DERMOSCOPY
AN ATLAS 3RD EDITION

SCOTT W. MENZIES, MB BS, PhD
Associate Professor, Discipline of Dermatology, Faculty of Medicine,
The University of Sydney and Director, Sydney Melanoma Diagnostic Centre,
Sydney Cancer Centre, Royal Prince Alfred Hospital, Sydney, Australia

KERRY A. CROTTY, MB BS, BSc(Med), FRCPA
Dermatologist, Sydney Melanoma Diagnostic Centre;
Dermatopathologist, Skin and Cancer Foundation Australia

CHRISTIAN INGVAR, MD, PhD
Associate Professor, Department of Surgery, Lund University Hospital,
Lund, Sweden

WILLIAM H. McCARTHY, MB BS, MEd, FRACS
Emeritus Professor of Surgery (Melanoma and Skin Oncology),
The University of Sydney

The McGraw·Hill Companies

Sydney New York San Francisco Auckland
Bangkok Bogotá Caracas Hong Kong
Kuala Lumpur Lisbon London Madrid
Mexico City Milan New Delhi San Juan
Seoul Singapore Taipei Toronto

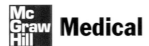
Medical

The **McGraw-Hill** Companies

First published 1996
Second edition 2003

Text and images © 2009 Scott Menzies, William H. McCarthy, Kerry Ann Crotty, Christian Ingvar
Design © 2009 McGraw-Hill Australia Pty Ltd
Additional owners of copyright are acknowledged in on-page credits.
Every effort has been made to trace and acknowledge copyrighted material. The authors and publishers tender their apologies should any infringement have occurred.

National Library of Australia Cataloguing-in-Publication Data

Author:	Menzies, Scott W. (Scott Whitton)
Title:	Dermoscopy: an atlas / Scott Menzies.
Edition:	3rd ed.
ISBN:	9780070159099 (pbk.)
Notes:	Includes index.
	Bibliography.
Subjects:	Dermatology—Atlases.
	Medical microscopy.
	Pigmentation disorders—Atlases.
	Melanoma—Atlases.

Dewey Number: 616.50758

Published in Australia by
McGraw-Hill Australia Pty Ltd
Level 2, 82 Waterloo Road, North Ryde NSW 2113
Acquisitions editor: Elizabeth Walton
Production editor: Natalie Crouch
Editor: Nicole McKenzie
Proofreader: Ron Buck
Indexer: Jon Jermey
Art director: Astred Hicks
Cover Designer: Peta Nugent
Internal Designer: Natalie Bowra
Image preparation: Vision Graphics
Typeset in 10/14 pt Bembo by Midland Typesetters, Australia
Printed in China on 113 gsm matt art by 1010 Printing International Ltd

DERMOSCOPY
AN ATLAS

DEDICATION

This book is dedicated to our patients.

CONTENTS

PREFACE

The aim of this book is to give the reader (expert and non-expert) a comprehensive understanding of the role of dermoscopy for the diagnosis of skin tumors. There has been a considerable rewrite to this edition, reflecting the dramatic increase in the dermoscopy literature in the last six years. In addition, in an attempt to expose the reader to the full spectrum of morphological variety seen with the various lesion types and features, we have included 193 new figures. Chapter 1 (Introduction), with four new figures, now has a section on the expanded evidence for the use of dermoscopy in improving diagnostic accuracy and differences between glass-plate and cross-polarized devices. Chapter 2 (Diagnostic features), with 29 new figures, has new sections on the variety of recently described vessel types, target globules, and network, peripheral light-brown structureless areas, fat fingers, white network, and nevus morphology. Chapter 3 (Benign macules), with 7 new figures, has a further section on non-pigmented actinic keratoses. Chapter 4 (Melanocytic nevi) has a major rewrite with 57 new figures and new sections on global patterns of nevi, congenital, halo and recurrent nevi, and a significant extension of the section on acral nevi. Chapter 5 (Melanoma), with 44 new figures, also has a major rewrite with a new section on amelanotic/hypomelanotic melanoma and substantial extensions to the sections on in situ melanoma, subungual melanoma, and all its differential diagnoses and cutaneous melanoma metastases. Chapter 6 (Non-melanocytic tumors), with 25 new figures, has new sections on Bowen's disease and clear cell acanthoma, additional observations on seborrheic keratoses and hemangioma, and an extensive rewrite of the section on dermatofibromas. Chapter 7 (Two-step procedure for diagnosis) includes more detailed descriptions of exceptions to the rules. In contrast to the CD-ROM found in the second edition, we have developed a website to illustrate cases using the two-step procedure. This has the advantage of allowing additional cases to be included over time. Chapter 8 (Computerized monitoring), with 14 new figures, has been rewritten to allow the incorporation of new literature on both short- and long-term digital monitoring. Finally, we have a new Chapter 9 (Summary), which uses 13 new schematic figures to summarize the diagnostic features of the main lesions.

Like previous editions, two main magnifications of the dermoscopy photographs have been used in this book. The small (85 × 54 mm) photographs are at a magnification of ×6.5. With some lesions, the full ×10 magnification is required to adequately discern certain features, resulting in the large (140 × 90 mm) photographs. For computerized monitoring photographs the magnification is indicated in Figure 8.2a.

ACKNOWLEDGMENTS

The authors wish to thank the staff of the Sydney Melanoma Diagnostic Centre and the Anatomical Pathology Department of Royal Prince Alfred Hospital. In particular we thank Michelle Avramidis and Betty Doan Tran who maintain the dermoscopy photographic database and Dr Malene Vestergaard who helped with the online quiz. We also thank Dr Harold Rabinovitz, Dr Graham Mason, Dr Luc Thomas, Dr Giuseppe Argenziano, Dr Maria Pizzichetta, Dr Alan Cameron, Dr Riccardo Bono, and Dr Ignazio Stanganelli for supplying some photographs of important figures without which this atlas would be incomplete.

CHAPTER ONE

INTRODUCTION

In *vivo* cutaneous surface microscopy, epiluminescence microscopy, dermatoscopy, magnified oil immersion diascopy, and dermoscopy are terms that describe the use of an incident light magnification system to examine cutaneous lesions, usually with liquid at the skin–microscope interface.[1] Currently the internationally accepted term is "dermoscopy". The use of liquid or polarized filters removes the normal scattering of light at the stratum corneum, thus allowing the epidermis to become translucent. This permits a detailed examination of the pigmented structures of the epidermis and dermoepidermal junction.[2,3] The early studies of surface microscopy of the skin by Hinselmann[4] and Goldman[5,6] were not expanded to any great extent until the regular use of oil immersion.[2,3,7] Since then, dermoscopy has been shown to greatly enhance the clinical diagnosis of nearly all pigmented skin tumors.[8–29] However, its main impact has been to improve the diagnostic accuracy of melanoma compared to naked eye examination.[30]

In a recent meta-analysis performed exclusively in studies in a clinical setting, the diagnostic odds ratio (the best measure for diagnostic accuracy) for melanoma using dermoscopy was 15.6 times higher compared with naked eye examination.[31] The overall estimate of sensitivity (percentage of melanomas correctly diagnosed) was higher for dermoscopy (90%) than for eye examination alone (71%). While there was no statistical evidence of a difference in specificity for melanoma (percentage of non-melanomas correctly diagnosed) between dermoscopy (90%) and eye examination (81%), a dramatic effect of dermoscopy on specificity is best examined by its effect on excision rates. In a randomized trial in a specialist setting of naked eye versus naked eye and dermoscopy examination there was a significant 42% reduction in patients referred to biopsy in the dermoscopy arm.[29] This is consistent with the retrospective findings of a significant reduction of the benign/malignant ratio of excised melanocytic lesions in clinicians trained in the use of dermoscopy from 18:1 (pre-dermoscopy era)

to 4:1 (post-dermoscopy era).[32] In contrast, non-users of dermoscopy continued their diagnostic performance without improvement (from 12:1 to 14:1).

So the evidence is plentiful that dermoscopy decreases the need for biopsy *in addition* to improving the detection of melanoma compared with naked eye examination. This is perhaps best expressed by its corollary: that naked eye examination may miss detecting melanoma while also leading to needless excisions. *We have published work showing a 39% improvement in the sensitivity for the diagnosis of melanoma using this Atlas (first edition) as the basis of an education intervention for primary care physicians.*[18] *The second edition formed the basis of the education intervention that led to a reduction of more than 50% in excisions or referrals of pigmented skin lesions in a clinical trial with primary care physicians.*[33]

Groups have used magnifications from ×6 to ×400.[2,3,34–39] To achieve this range of magnification, large, and expensive binocular microscopes are required. Inexpensive hand-held instruments (e.g. Dermatoscope—Heine Ltd; Dermlite-3Gen,LLC) have been developed which allow a fixed magnification of ×10 and this is now the favored magnification.[40] It should be emphasized that dermoscopy using non-glass plate polarizing filtered devices can be significantly different to those of liquid-glass plate devices.[41] In the former, structures such as milia-like cysts, crypts, multiple blue-gray dots and blue-white veil may not be visualized. In contrast compression using glass plate devices may decrease the visualization of vessels and white streaks. Unless specified, all dermoscopy photographs presented here were achieved using the liquid-glass plate technique. In regards to these devices, the more recent models using greater illumination with LED light sources has improved the range of colors and structures detected.[42] Finally, we routinely use 70% ethanol which provides superior visualization in addition to antisepsis between patient use.[43–45]

References

1. Cohen, D, Sangueza, O, Fass, E, Stiller, M. In vivo cutaneous surface microscopy: revised nomenclature. *Int J Dermatol* 1993; 32: 257–8.

2. MacKie, R. An aid to the preoperative assessment of pigmented lesions of the skin. *Br J Dermatol* 1971; 85: 232–8.

3. Fritsch, P, Pechlaner, R. Differentiation of benign from malignant melanocytic lesions using incident light microscopy. In: Ackerman A. (ed.). *Pathology of malignant melanoma.* New York, Masson, 1981; 301–12.

4. Hinselmann, H. Die Bedeutung der Kolposkopie fur den Dermatologen. *Dermat Wchnschr* 1933; 96: 533–43.

5. Goldman, L, Younker, W. Studies in microscopy of the surface of the skin. *J Invest Dermatol* 1947; 9: 11–16.

6. Goldman, L. Some investigative studies of pigmented nevi with cutaneous microscopy. *J Invest Dermatol* 1951; 16: 407–27.

7. Fritsch, P, Pechlaner, R. The pigmented network: A new tool for the diagnosis of pigmented lesions. *J Invest Dermatol* 1980; 74: 458–9.

8. Steiner, A, Pehamberger, H, Wolff, K. In vivo epiluminescence microscopy of pigmented skin lesions. II Diagnosis of small pigmented skin lesions and early detection of malignant melanoma. *J Am Acad Dermatol* 1987; 17: 584–91.

9. Pehamberger, H, Binder, M, Steiner, A, Wolff, K. In vivo epiluminescence microscopy: Improvement of early diagnosis of melanoma. *J Invest Dermatol* 1993; 100: 356S–62S.

10. Nachbar, F, Stolz, W, Merkle, T, et al. The ABCD rule of dermatoscopy. *J Am Acad Dermatol* 1994; 30: 551–9.

11. Krahn, G, Gottlober, P, Sander, C, Peter, RU. Dermatoscopy and high frequency sonography: Two useful non-invasive methods to increase preoperative diagnostic accuracy in pigmented skin lesions. *Pigment Cell Res* 1998; 11: 151–4.

12. Steiner, A, Pehamberger, H, Binder, M, Wolff, K. Pigmented Spitz nevi: Improvement of the diagnostic accuracy by epiluminescence microscopy. *J Am Acad Dermatol* 1992; 27: 697–701.

13. Binder, M, Schwarz, M, Winkler, A, et al. Epiluminescence microscopy: A useful tool for the diagnosis of pigmented skin lesions for formally trained dermatologists. *Arch Dermatol* 1995; 131: 286–91.

14. Pazzini, C, Pozzi, M, Betti, R, et al. Improvement of diagnostic accuracy in the clinical diagnosis of pigmented skin lesions by epiluminescence microscopy. *Skin Cancer* 1996; 11: 159–61.

15. Binder, M, Puespoeck-Schwarz, M, Steiner, A, et al. Epiluminescence microscopy of small pigmented skin lesions: Short-term formal training improves the diagnostic performance of dermatologists. *J Am Acad Dermatol* 1997; 36: 197–202.

16. Carli, P, De Giorgi, V, Naldi, L, Dosi, G. Reliability and inter-observer agreement of dermoscopic diagnosis of melanoma and melanocytic naevi. *European J Cancer Prev* 1998; 7: 397–402.

17. Stanganelli, I, Serafini, M, Cainelli, T, et al. Accuracy of epiluminescence microscopy among practical dermatologists: a study from the Emilia-Romagna region of Italy. *Tumori* 1998; 84: 701–5.

18. Westerhoff, K, McCarthy, WH, Menzies, SW. Increase in the sensitivity for melanoma diagnosis by primary care physicians using skin surface microscopy. *Br J Dermatol* 2000; 143: 1016–20.

19. Bafounta, M, Beauchet, A, Aegerter, P, Saiag, P. Is dermoscopy (epiluminescence microscopy) useful for the diagnosis of melanoma? Results of a meta-analysis using techniques adapted to the evaluation of diagnostic tests. *Arch Dermatol* 2001; 137: 1361–3.

20. Kittler, H, Pehamberger, H, Wolff, K, et al. Diagnostic accuracy of dermoscopy. *Lancet Oncology* 2002; 3:159–65.

21. Stanganelli, I, Serafini, M, Bucch, L. A cancer-registry-assisted evaluation of the accuracy of digital epiluminescence microscopy associated with clinical examination of pigmented skin lesions. *Dermatology* 2000; 200: 11–6.

22. Benelli, C, Roscetti, E, Dal Pozzo, V, et al. The dermoscopic versus the clinical diagnosis of melanoma. *Eur J Dermatol* 1999; 9: 470–6.

23. Dummer, W, Doehnel, KA, Remy, W. Videomicroscopy in differential diagnosis of skin tumors and secondary prevention of malignant melanoma. *Hautarzt* 1993; 44: 772–6.

24. Cristofolini, M, Zumiani, G, Bauer, P, et al. Dermatoscopy: usefulness in the differential diagnosis

of cutaneous pigmentary lesions. *Melanoma Res* 1994; 4: 391–4.

25. Carli, P, Mannone, F, De Giorgi, V, et al. The problem of false-positive diagnosis in melanoma screening: the impact of dermoscopy. *Melanoma Res* 2003; 13: 179–82.

26. Bono, A, Tolomio, E, Trincone, S, et al. Micro-melanoma detection: a clinical study on 206 consecutive cases of pigmented skin lesions with a diameter < or = 3 mm. *Br J Dermatol* 2006; 155: 570–3.

27. Bono, A, Bartoli, C, Cascinelli, N, et al. Melanoma detection. A prospective study comparing diagnosis with the naked eye, dermatoscopy and telespectrophotometry. *Dermatology* 2002; 205: 362–6.

28. Argenziano, G, Puig, S, Zalaudek, I, et al. Dermoscopy improves accuracy of primary care physicians to triage lesions suggestive of skin cancer. *J Clin Oncol* 2006; 24: 1877–82.

29. Carli, P, de Giorgi, V, Chiarugi, A, et al. Addition of dermoscopy to conventional naked-eye examination in melanoma screening: a randomized study. *J Am Acad Dermatol* 2004; 50: 683–9.

30. Menzies, SW, Zalaudek, I. Why perform dermoscopy? The evidence for its role in the routine management of pigmented skin lesions. *Arch Dermatol* 2006; 142: 1211–2.

31. Vestergaard, ME, Macaskill, P, Holt PE, Menzies, SW. Dermoscopy compared with naked eye examination for the diagnosis of primary melanoma: a meta-analysis of studies performed in a clinical setting. *Br J Dermatol* 2008; 159: 669–76.

32. Carli, P, De Giorgi, V, Crocetti, E, et al. Improvement of malignant/benign ratio in excised melanocytic lesions in the "dermoscopy era": a retrospective study 1997–2001. *Br J Dermatol* 2004; 150: 687–92.

33. Menzies, SW, et al. Manuscript submitted.

34. Menzies, S, Crotty, K, McCarthy, W. The morphologic criteria of the pseudopod in surface microscopy. *Arch Dermatol* 1995; 131: 436–40.

35. Soyer, H, Smolle, J, Hodl, S, Pachernegg, H, Kerl, H. Surface microscopy. A new approach to the diagnosis of cutaneous pigmented tumors. *Am J Dermatopath* 1989; 11: 1–10.

36. Kreusch, J, Rassner, G. Strukturanalyse melanozytischer pigmentmale durch auflichtmikroskopie. *Hautarzt* 1990; 41: 27–33.

37. Pehamberger, H, Steiner, A, Wolff, K. In vivo epiluminescence microscopy of pigmented skin lesions. I. Pattern analysis of pigmented skin lesions. *J Am Acad Dermatol* 1987; 17: 571–83.

38. Kenet, R, Kang, S, Kenet, B, Fitzpatrick, T, Sober, A, Barnhill, R. Clinical diagnosis of pigmented lesions using digital epiluminescence microscopy. *Arch Dermatol* 1993; 129: 157–74.

39. Puppin, D, Salomon, D, Saurat, J. Amplified surface microscopy. *J Am Acad Dermatol* 1993; 28: 923–7.

40. Braun-Falco, O, Stolz, W, Bilek, P, et al. Das Dermatoskop: eine Vereinfachung der Auflichtmikroskopie von pigmentierten Hautveranderungen. *Hautarzt* 1990; 41: 131–6.

41. Benvenuto-Andrade, C, Dusza, SW, Agero, AL, et al. Differences between polarized light dermoscopy and immersion contact dermoscopy for the evaluation of skin lesions. *Arch Dermatol* 2007; 143: 329–38.

42. Blum, A, Jaworski, S. Clear differences in hand-held dermoscopes. *J Dtsch Dermatol Ges* 2006; 4: 1054–7.

43. Gewirtzman, AJ, Saurat, JH, Braun, RP. An evaluation of dermoscopy fluids and application techniques. *Br J Dermatol* 2003; 149: 59–63.

44. Kelly, SC, Purcell, SM. Prevention of nosocomial infection during dermoscopy? *Dermatol Surg* 2006; 32: 552–5.

45. Hausermann, P, Widmer, A, Itin, P. Dermatoscope as vector for transmissible diseases—no apparent risk of nosocomial infections in outpatients. *Dermatology* 2006; 212: 27–30.

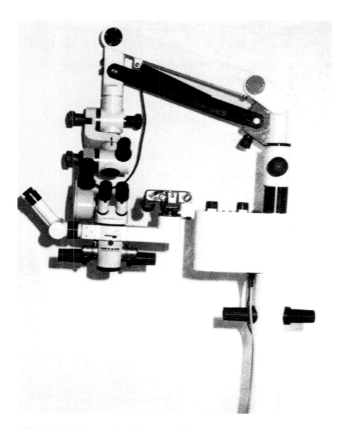

FIGURE 1.1 Binocular microscope*

The initial instruments used in the investigation of surface microscopy were binocular microscopes. These have the advantage of allowing a greater range of magnification (in this case ×6 to ×40) but are expensive and cumbersome.

This figure is from: Pehamberger, H, Steiner, A, Wolff, K. In vivo epiluminescence microscopy of pigmented skin lesions. I. Pattern analysis of pigmented skin lesions. J Am Acad Dermatol 1987; 17: 571–83.

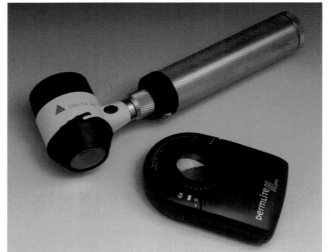

FIGURE 1.2 Hand-held surface microscopes

With the introduction of the hand-held surface microscopes in the late 1980s, cutaneous surface microscopy became an inexpensive method of improving the diagnosis of nearly all pigmented skin lesions. These instruments have a fixed magnification of ×10. Devices can use either the liquid/glass plate technique or polarized filters without glass plate compression. In regards to the liquid/glass plate devices, the more recent models that use greater illumination with LED light sources has improved the range of colors and structures detected.

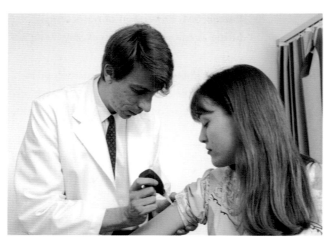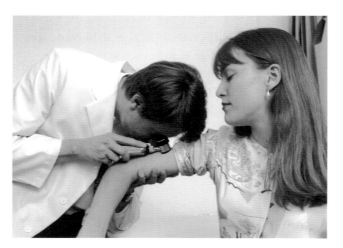

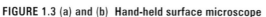

FIGURE 1.3 (a) and (b) Hand-held surface microscope

Oil or liquid (e.g. mineral oil, immersion oil, liquid paraffin, ultrasound gel, clear antiseptic solution, 70% ethanol) is applied to the lesion prior to examination (a). We routinely use 70% ethanol which provides superior visualisation in addition to antisepsis between patient use. The surface microscope is then placed directly against the skin and focused (b).

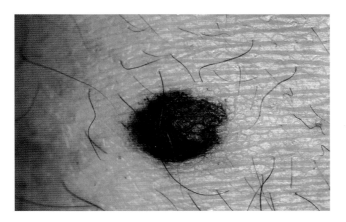

FIGURE 1.4 (a) Clinical view
Clinically this pigmented lesion is relatively structureless.

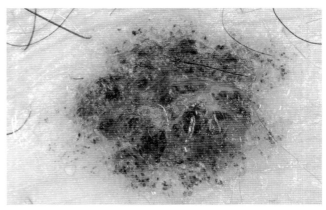

FIGURE 1.4 (b) Dermoscopy view without oil application
The simple magnification by ×10 improves the definition of this lesion remarkably. However, reflection of light from the stratum corneum distorts the view, resulting in poor detail of the underlying structure.

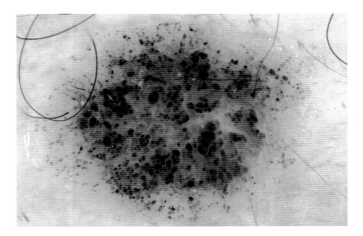

FIGURE 1.4 (c) Dermoscopy view with oil application
The addition of liquid to the surface prevents the random scatter of light at the stratum corneum–air interface. This essentially makes the non-pigmented epidermis "invisible" and allows the pigmented structures of the epidermis, dermoepidermal junction and dermis to be seen. The result is a technique that enables characterization of more than 100 morphological features of pigmented lesions.

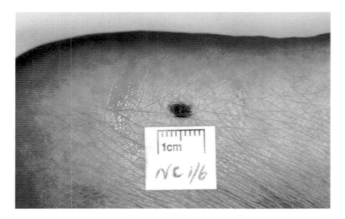

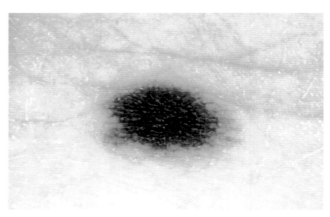

FIGURE 1.5 (a) Clinical view

FIGURE 1.5 (b) Dermoscopy view without oil application

FIGURE 1.5 (c) Dermoscopy view with oil application

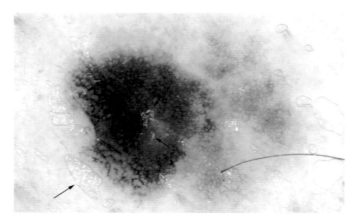

FIGURE 1.6 Artefacts

Air bubbles (large arrow) are a commonly seen artefact in dermoscopy. They are due to an inadequate application of liquid, but are often unavoidable if a lesion has an irregularly contoured surface. In some images a white photographic artefact (small arrow) may be seen.

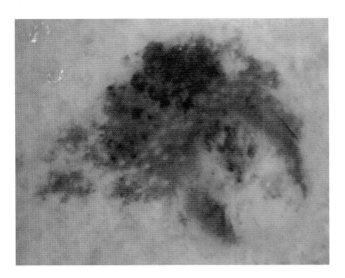

FIGURE 1.7 (a) Liquid/glass plate dermoscopy view

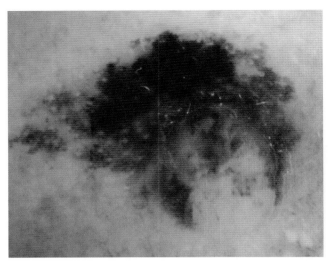

FIGURE 1.7 (b) Cross polarized non-compression dermoscopy view

Note the almost complete loss of blue-white veil in this invasive melanoma. In addition, melanin appears darker.

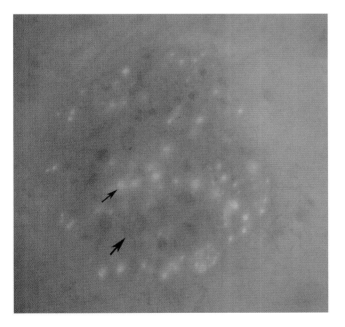

FIGURE 1.8 (a) Liquid/glass plate dermoscopy view

FIGURE 1.8 (b) Cross polarized non-compression dermoscopy view

Here milia-like cysts (small arrow in (a)) are not visualized and irregular crypts (large arrow in (a)) are less visualized compared with the liquid/glass plate instrument.

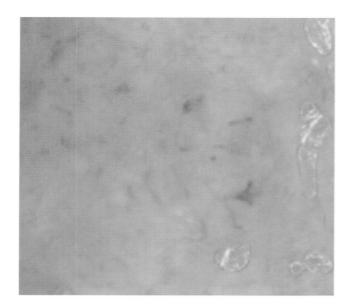

FIGURE 1.9 (a) Liquid/glass plate dermoscopy view

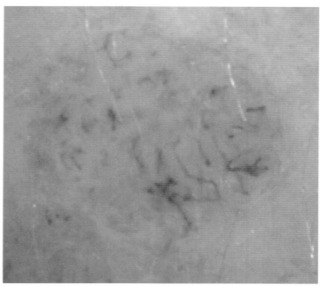

FIGURE 1.9 (b) Cross polarized non-compression dermoscopy view

Lack of compression of the lesion with the glass plate increases the visualization of vessels and changes the morphology of vessel structures.

CHAPTER TWO

THE DIAGNOSTIC FEATURES OF DERMOSCOPY

Unaided visualization of pigmented skin lesions in the clinical setting is limited in that only a few morphological features can be identified. However, dermoscopy allows the identification of over one hundred features. The diagnosis of pigmented skin lesions using dermoscopy requires each of these features to be individually distinguished, and the important diagnostic features are defined in this chapter. Where possible, the consensus terminology described elsewhere[1–3] is observed.

Each feature will have a specificity and sensitivity for a particular diagnosis. The **specificity** is equal to the number of scored negatives divided by the total number of lesions *without* that diagnosis, expressed as a percentage. The **sensitivity** of a variable is equal to the number of scored positives of that variable divided by the total number of lesions with that diagnosis, expressed as a percentage. For example, the feature of blue–white veil has a specificity of 97% and a sensitivity of 51% for invasive melanoma. This signifies that 51% of invasive melanomas have blue–white veil, while only 3% of non-melanomas have this feature.

Pigmentation

The pigmentation observed in dermoscopy primarily involves two forms, hemoglobin (vasculature) and melanin. Vasculature is seen either as the color red (in diffuse erythema, telangiectasia, or some cases of lacunes in hemangiomas), or red-blue, which occurs in the remainder of hemangioma lacunes. In the case of melanin, the color seen in dermoscopy depends on its depth in the skin. At the stratum corneum melanin appears black, at the dermoepidermal junction it appears brown and at the dermis it appears as gray or blue (Figure 2.1). Histopathologically, melanin can be seen in melanocytes or melanocyte-derived cells (nevus cells, melanoma), keratinocytes of the epidermis, macrophages in the dermis (melanophages) or sequestered in various tumor cells (e.g. pigmented basal cell carcinoma).

The presence of **multiple colors** in a lesion observed under dermoscopy is a highly significant feature of invasive melanoma.[4–6] When graded for the 6 colors of tan, dark brown, blue, gray, black, and red/blue, the presence of **5–6 colors** has a specificity of 92% and a sensitivity of 53% for invasive melanoma (Figures 2.2–2.3).[4]

Conversely, a **single color** rarely, if ever, occurs in invasive pigmented melanoma.[4,7]

Symmetrical pigmentation pattern refers to symmetry of pattern/texture along *all* axes through the center (of gravity) of a lesion (Figures 2.25–2.29). It does *not* require symmetry of shape. Nearly all invasive melanomas lack symmetry of pigmentation (**asymmetric pigmentation pattern**) (Figures 2.30–2.33), while the presence of symmetrical pigmentation is often the defining feature of benign pigmented lesions.[4,7] While asymmetric pigmentation pattern is found in the vast majority of invasive melanomas, 54% of atypical pigmented non-melanomas also have this feature.

Eccentric hyperpigmentation is seen as increased focal pigmentation at the edge of a lesion. While it is a significant feature of melanoma overall, when found in melanocytic nevi lacking other specific dermoscopic features of melanoma it is not indicative of malignancy.[8]

Blue-white veil

The terms "whitish veil" and "milky way" refer to the dermoscopic feature of a white "ground glass" appearance. This is seen when compact orthokeratosis, with or without hypergranulosis, is present.[1,9,10] "Gray-blue veil" or "areas" refer to an ill-defined, usually irregular bluish or blue-gray area. Histopathologically this corresponds to superficial fibrosis with melanophages and/or pigmented malignant cells in the papillary dermis.[1,11] It has also been referred to as the presence of blue pigment in a whitish veil.[10] Because of this, clinicians often use the terms milky way and blue-gray veil synonymously. Both have a high specificity for melanoma, but are sometimes seen in angiomas or pigmented BCCs. For these reasons, the authors have defined *blue-white veil* as *an irregular, indistinct, confluent blue pigment with an overlying white ground-glass film, not associated with red-blue lacunes.*[4]

As also confirmed by others[12], blue-white veil represents histologically the presence of a compact aggregation of heavily pigmented cells (usually melanoma and/or melanophages) in the dermis in combination with compact orthokeratosis (compact, thickened stratum corneum). Its dermoscopic appearance can be differentiated from multiple blue dots (scattered dermal melanophages) because of its confluence of pigment (versus a speckled pattern seen in multiple blue dots); from red-blue lacunes, ovoid nests, and leaf-like areas because of their distinct shapes (versus the irregular indistinct shape of blue-white veil); and from the uniform steel-blue color seen in blue nevi because of the irregular non-uniform nature of blue-white veil. Under this definition, the blue-white veil has a specificity of 97% and a sensitivity of 51% for invasive melanoma and is the most significant diagnostic feature of hypomelanotic melanoma (Figures 2.34–2.42).[4,13]

Dots and globules

Accumulation of pigment into round or oval dots and globules is seen in many pigmented lesions. Their color is determined by the level of the pigment in the skin. Dots and globules are distinguished only by their size (a globule being a large dot) and therefore are usually considered together. The exception are the features of multiple brown dots and multiple blue-gray dots, where globules are excluded in these definitions, and multiple peripheral brown globules and multiple blue-gray globules, where dots are excluded.

Black dots/globules represent localized pigment accumulation (often melanoma cells) in the stratum corneum.[9,14,15] They can be found in benign pigmented lesions, but tend to be central in position. While they are a significant finding in any position in a lesion, they are more specific for melanoma when found peripherally (defining the edge of the lesion or lying within the body of the lesion near the edge) (Figures 2.43–2.47).[4,14,16]

TABLE 2.1 Black dots/globules: sensitivity and specificity for invasive melanoma[4]

	Specificity (%)	Sensitivity (%)
Any position	81	60
Peripheral	92	42
Central	82	51

Multiple brown dots are seen as aggregations of well-defined dark brown dots that represent supra-basal (intraepidermal) collections of pigment, usually melanoma cells. They are a highly significant feature of melanoma, with a specificity of 97% and a sensitivity of 30% for invasive melanoma (Figures 2.48–2.50).[4]

Brown dots/globules occur in many pigmented lesions and represent pigmented cell nests at or near the dermoepidermal junction.[1,9,11,14,15,17] In benign common nevi they are usually regular in size and distribution, in contrast to melanoma and dysplastic nevi, where they appear irregular in shape and distribution.[13,16] However, in one variant of dysplastic nevi, brown globules can be seen in a circumferential position defining the edge of the lesion. These are referred to as **multiple peripheral brown globules**.[18] In Spitz nevi they are often multiple, peripheral, and multilayered.[11,19] Using amplified surface microscopy,[17] brown globules in melanocytic-derived pigmented lesions can be classified according to the position of the globule in relation to the melanocytic network (rete ridge) (Figures 2.51–2.56).

Multiple blue-gray dots are seen as diffuse, partly aggregated dots, often described as "pepper-like" in morphology. Histopathologically they are melanophages in the dermis.[15,20] Melanophages are melanin-laden macrophages that are particularly seen in regression of pigmented lesions (although their presence does not always indicate regression). Since histopathological regression is a common feature of malignant melanoma,[21] the presence of multiple blue-gray dots is a significant feature of melanoma, with a specificity of 91% and a sensitivity of 45% for invasive melanoma.[4] While multiple blue-gray dots (granularity) is a significant feature of melanoma, dysplastic nevi do not require excision when they have small focal areas (<10% of the lesion surface area) of multiple blue-gray dots without other dermoscopic features of melanoma.[23,25] (Figures 2.59–2.63).

Multiple blue-gray globules should be differentiated from multiple blue-gray dots by their larger size and better circumscribed morphology. They are a highly specific feature (97%) for pigmented BCC and represent melanin in the dermal tumor nests (in melanocytes, tumor cells, or stroma)[26,36] (Figures 2.135–2.137). They can also be seen in a rare variant of pigmented seborrheic keratoses (Figures 6.35–6.36).

Target globules are seen as brown to blue globules with a surrounding white halo. They are found more frequently in congenital nevi (Figure 2.139).[27–29]

Pseudopods

The pseudopod (Greek: *pseudos*—"false", *podos*—"foot") is a dermoscopic feature that represents the radial growth phase of melanoma. Histopathologically pseudopods are intraepidermal or junctional, confluent radial nests of melanoma.[15,18] Dermoscopically they are bulbous and often kinked projections seen at the edge of superficial spreading melanomas. Their color ranges from tan to black, but they tend to be heavily pigmented. They are often seen at the end of radial streaming, but can occur directly from the tumor edge, often not associated with the pigmented network. Unlike in some Spitz nevi, pseudopods never appear around the circumference of a melanoma, instead they are irregularly or focally present at their edge. Because of their morphological variation, a strict definition has been proposed (see Figure 2.64).[18] With this definition, the pseudopod has a specificity of 97% and a sensitivity of 23% for invasive melanoma (Figures 2.64–2.74).

Radial streaming

Like the pseudopod, radial streaming represents histopathologically the radial growth phase of melanoma. While histologically identical to the pseudopod, their dermoscopic morphology is different and they should therefore be considered under separate definitions.

They appear as radially and asymmetrically arranged parallel linear extensions at the edge of the tumor. While they can occur within the body of a melanoma, they are a specific feature of melanoma only when seen at the edge. Under this definition, radial streaming has a specificity of 96% and a sensitivity of 18% for invasive melanoma (Figures 2.75–2.79).[4]

Pigmented network

The pigmented network is the unifying dermoscopic feature of melanocytic-derived lesions (ephelis, lentigo, junctional and compound nevi, and melanoma).[9,15,22] It is formed by melanocytes, melanin in basal keratinocytes or melanocyte-derived cells at the basal layer of the epidermis. When viewed vertically with the surface microscope, these cells produce areas of dense pigment which are due to projections of the rete pegs/ridges (constituting the grids or "cords" of the network), and areas of relatively little pigment, which are due to the projections of the dermal papillae (constituting the holes of the network) (Figures 2.4–2.9).

While the pigmented network usually signifies a lesion is melanocyte-derived, it is not found in every melanocyte-derived lesion. For example, only 59% of invasive melanomas have a network.[4]

A discrete (lightly pigmented) network that also has a regular width of the cords making up the net (**discrete/regular network**) is generally found in benign melanocytic lesions (lentigo, junctional, and compound nevi).[16] A discrete/regular network is found only in 7% of melanomas, and is a significant negative correlate of melanoma (Figure 2.17).[4] Because of increased basal pigmentation in many dermatofibromas, 72% of these lesions have a discrete delicate network.[50]

A prominent (darkly pigmented) network with irregular-width cords (**prominent/irregular network**) is often found in dysplastic nevi, Spitz nevi, and in in situ and invasive melanoma. However, using the low power magnification of the hand-held surface microscopes, a prominent/irregular network is not a statistically significant feature of invasive melanoma (Figure 2.18).[4,6]

A network with broad-width cords (**broadened network**) is a significant finding of melanoma. While it is the commonest feature of lentigo maligna, it also has specificity for invasive melanoma (specificity 86% and sensitivity 35%) (Figures 2.19–2.20).[4] The broadened network of lentigo maligna (Hutchinson's melanotic freckle) on the face can form dark (brown to black) **rhomboidal structures**.[24] These occur in 49% of lentigo maligna but are absent in the majority of benign pigmented macules of the face (Figure 2.21). Finally, in pigmented lesions of the face, follicular openings can create a **pseudo-broadened network**. This can occur in both melanocytic and non-melanocytic lesions (Figures 2.23–2.24).

A variant of the network pattern is the **target network**. Here, target globules are surrounded by a normal pigment network. This feature is found more frequently in congenital nevi (Figure 2.140).[27–29]

Pigment network on the palms and soles

The pigment network on volar sites (palms or soles) has a distinct morphology that differs from nevi on non-volar body sites. While a number of variations have been described, the basic element of acral nevi is the **parallel furrow pattern**. The histopathological correlation of this is nevus cells found in the crista profunda limitans, an epidermal rete ridge underlying the surface furrow.[30] Melanin is found in a column from this rete ridge to and including the stratum corneum.[31–33] This vertical column gives the dermoscopy appearance of the parallel furrows of the skin surface markings being preferentially pigmented. Depending upon the anatomical site on the sole of the foot the parallel furrow pattern may remain intact (non-arch of the foot), show a **lattice-like pattern** (arch of the foot) with pigmentation on the furrows and lines crossing the furrows, or a **fibrillar/filamentous pattern** with a mesh-like or delicate filamentous pigmentation crossing the lines of skin markings due to slanting of the columns on the weight bearing surface of the sole (Figures 2.11–2.14).

On volar sites the **parallel ridge pattern** has a sensitivity of 86% and specificity of 99% for the diagnosis of melanoma (both invasive and in situ).[34] Here the broader ridges (in contrast to the furrows) of the surface skin markings are predominantly pigmented (Figures 2.15–2.16).

Negative pigment network

A negative pigment network is seen as a "negative" of the pigmented network, with light areas making up the cords of the network and dark areas filling the "holes". Histopathologically it represents elongated hypomelanotic rete ridges. It is seen in many Spitz nevi.[35] However, the negative pigment network is also a highly specific feature of invasive melanoma (95% specificity, 22% sensitivity)[4] and also occurs in dysplastic nevi. For this reason, the presence of a negative pigment network should not be used as the only feature to diagnose Spitz nevi (Figures 2.80–2.83).

The lesion edge and shape

The edge of the pigmented lesion has been shown to contain many of the important diagnostic features in dermoscopy. As well as specific features such as pseudopods, radial streaming, dots/globules, and depigmentation, the general characteristic of the edge also gives important diagnostic information. An **irregular edge** is seen in 94% of melanomas, but it is also seen in 64% of other pigmented lesions. An edge showing sharp contrast with the normal skin (**abrupt edge**), in *any part* of the lesion, is a feature of melanoma. This is particularly seen with an abrupt edge of the pigmented network. The network classically graduates into the normal skin of benign nevi. While 77% of melanomas have some part of their edge ending abruptly, 33% of non-melanomas also have this feature.[4]

The **moth-eaten** edge is seen as well-defined "punched-out", concave areas at the edge of a lesion. While it is a common feature of the ephelis (freckle), it can occasionally be seen in the lentigo, flat seborrheic keratoses, and lentigo maligna (Figure 2.85).

Regular shape refers to a lesion that approximates shape symmetry along both its axes. It is a highly negative correlate of invasive melanoma, with only 3% of melanomas having this feature. In contrast, 50% of non-melanomas approximate regular shape.[4]

The vasculature

Erythema is seen as diffuse, pink-red, poorly demarcated areas. It is a significant finding in invasive melanoma, with a sensitivity of 68% and a specificity of 72%.[4] However, in any irritated lesion, erythema can be seen. Furthermore, erythema is common in dysplastic nevi.[37] A variant of erythema is **milky red areas**.[13,37,39,40] Here, erythema with an overlying milky film-like area has a sensitivity of 51% and specificity of 71% for amelanotic/hypomelanotic melanoma (Figure 2.105).[13] Finally, **more than one shade of pink** color is also a feature of amelanotic/hypomelanotic melanoma (32% sensitivity, 83% specificity) (Figure 2.105).[13]

Telangiectasia are more readily seen with dermoscopy. They represent dilated vessels in the papillary dermis. Telangiectasia occur in 73% of BCCs.[36] Fifty percent of invasive melanomas have telangiectasia.[4] The most significant vascular feature of amelanotic/hypomelanotic melanoma are telangiectasia found predominantly in a central versus peripheral position (**predominant central vessels**). This feature has a 16% sensitivity and 94% specificity for amelanotic/hypomelanotic melanoma (Figure 2.106).[13] The morphology of telangiectasia can be helpful in distinguishing lesions. **Arborizing (tree-like) telangiectasia** with distinct branching of the vessels and **large diameter telangiectasia** both are a significant finding in pigmented BCC.[36,37] Arborizing vessels are found in 52% of pigmented BCC, 23% of melanoma and 8% of benign pigmented lesions (Figures 2.92–2.93).[36] Only 9% of amelanotic/hypomelanotic melanomas have arborising vessels as the predominant vessel type.[13]

Dotted (pinpoint) vessels are found in melanocytic tumors[37] and occur in the same frequency in nevi and melanomas (Figures 2.86–2.87).[13] Larger dotted vessels giving the appearance of the capillaries of the renal glomerulus (**glomerular vessels**) are found in Bowen's disease, psoriatic plaques and clear cell acanthomas (Figure 2.88).[37,42–47] In clear cell acanthoma glomerular vessels may form a reticular-linear array or "**string of pearls**" pattern (Figure 2.89).

Comma vessels that appear "C" or comma shaped are found in 66% of dermal or congenital nevi and are highly specific for benign nevi.[37,39] Only 1% and 2.9% of amelanotic/

hypomelanotic melanomas have regularly distributed comma vessels and comma vessels as the predominant vessel type, respectively (Figures 2.90–2.91).[13]

Linear irregular vessels that are seen as irregular wave-like vessels without branching are a significant feature of melanoma particularly when they are the predominant vessel type (34% sensitivity and 80% specificity for amelanotic/hypomelanotic melanoma).[13,37,39] They are also a more specific feature of melanoma when found in combination with dotted vessels within a lesion (30% sensitivity and 85% specificity for amelanotic/hypomelanotic melanoma) (Figures 2.96–2.97).[13,37]

Hairpin vessels seen as twisting loops are the most frequent vessel found in keratinizing tumors (seborrhoeic keratosis, squamous cell carcinoma, keratoacanthoma) (Figures 2.94–2.95).[37] In keratinizing tumors hairpin vessels are often surrounded by a white halo (**halo vessels**) (Figures 2.98–2.99). However, when found in melanocytic tumors, hairpin vessels are a significant feature of melanoma, with 21% of amelanotic/hypomelanotic melanoma having hairpin vessels.[13]

Milky red globules seen as unfocussed red-pink globular structures are a significant feature of melanoma (Figure 2.104).[13,37,39,40] However, they are not present in a significantly different frequency between melanoma and benign melanocytic lesions.[13]

Crown vessels which are seen as orderly, bending, scarcely branching vessels disappearing at the centre of the lesion are found in sebaceous hyperplasia (Figure 2.100).[37] Finally, **winding (cork-screw) vessels** are more specifically found in cutaneous melanoma metastases (Figure 2.101).[41]

Red-blue lacunes are sharply demarcated, ovoid structures that may appear as red or red-blue in color. When many are present in a lesion, they are pathognomonic for hemangiomas. Dark to black lacunes are found in angiokeratoma or thrombosed hemangioma.[38] Histopathologically red-blue lacunes represent dilated vascular spaces in the dermis (Figures 2.102–2.103).

Leaf-like areas

Leaf-like areas are seen as brown to gray/blue, discrete, bulbous extensions arising almost exclusively in pigmented basal cell carcinomas (BCCs).[36] Histopathologically they represent nests of pigmented epithelial nodules of BCC.[1,26] They should be distinguished from pseudopods, because the bulbous projections of leaf-like areas are discrete pigmented nests, never arising from a network and usually not arising from a confluent pigmented tumor (Figures 2.107–2.108).[18,36]

Large blue-gray ovoid nests

Large blue-gray ovoid nests are well-circumscribed, confluent, or near confluent pigmented ovoid or elongated areas, larger than globules, and not intimately connected to a pigmented tumor body. They are the single most useful feature for the diagnosis of pigmented BCC, with 55% of pigmented BCC having this feature but only 3% of melanoma and 1% of benign pigmented lesions.[36] Again they are due to melanin in the dermal tumor nests (in melanocytes, tumor cells, or stroma)[26] (Figures 2.132–2.134).

Spoke wheel areas

Spoke wheel areas are well-circumscribed radial projections, usually tan but sometimes blue or gray, meeting at an often darker central axis. They are highly specific (100%) for pigmented BCC, but found in only 10% of these lesions (Figure 2.138).[36]

Ulceration

Ulceration occurs early in the evolution of BCC and late in invasive melanoma. It is found in 27% of pigmented BCC but only 13% of invasive melanoma and 1% of benign pigmented lesions. When found in the absence of a pigmented network it has significant specificity for the diagnosis of pigmented BCC (Figure 2.57).[36]

Milia-like cysts

Milia-like cysts are seen as discrete, white or yellow, opalescent, round bodies within the body of a lesion. Histopathologically they represent intraepidermal keratin cysts.[1] They are commonly seen in seborrheic keratoses, with multiple large milia-like cysts being almost pathognomonic for this lesion. They also are seen not uncommonly in compound or dermal nevi (particularly congenital nevi) and pigmented BCC. Solitary or a few milia-like cysts can occur in melanoma and rarely occur in other pigmented lesions. However, multiple milia-like cysts are rarely found in melanoma, with only 1% of amelanotic/hypomelanotic melanomas having four or more milia.[13] (Figures 2.109–2.111).

Keratin

The reason for using liquid on the skin in dermoscopy is that reflection of light from the stratum corneum is removed. Hence surface scale essentially disappears. However, when focally increased, scale (keratin) can be seen as a white or pale yellow crystalline (reflective) surface. It occurs commonly in pigmented solar keratoses and seborrheic keratoses, and is not infrequently found in melanoma (and less commonly in other melanocytic lesions) (Figure 2.112).

Fissures, ridges, and crypts

Fissures are seen as confluent branching clefts in the body of a lesion. In most cases they can be distinguished from the papillomatous clefts of compound or dermal nevi (**cobblestone pattern**) by their greater width. **Crypts** (comedo-like openings) appear as irregularly shaped craters. Fissures and crypts are seen primarily in seborrheic keratoses, but occur also in compound and dermal nevi (usually the congenital variety). Less commonly, fissures are found in melanoma and other pigmented lesions (Figures 2.113–2.119). The raised structures between fissures are called **ridges**. When ridges are enlarged or separated by larger width keratin filled fissures they can form linear, curvilinear, round/oval or branched "**fat fingers**" as seen in some pigmented seborrheic keratoses (Figure 2.115).[49]

Fingerprint-like structures

Light brown fingerprint-like structures can be found in solar lentigo or early flat seborrheic keratoses (which may arise from solar lentigo).[2,24] Fingerprint-like structures can be distinguished from a pigment network since the former has less net-like structures with finer compact light brown cords forming curvilinear structures (Figure 2.58).

Depigmentation

The finding of depigmentation may indicate histopatho-logical regression in pigmented lesions. It can also be found as a consequence of the absence of pigmented cells without regression (e.g. as seen in the dermal component of many melanocytic nevi and the amelanotic nodules of melanoma). Depigmentation found at any site within a lesion is a significant feature of invasive melanoma, but it lacks adequate specificity to be a clinically useful discriminant.[4] However, an irregular pattern of depigmentation (**irregular depigmentation**) is more specific,[4,6,16] with a specificity of 92% and a sensitivity of 46% for invasive melanoma (Figures 2.120–2.121).

A variety of irregular depigmentation is **scar-like depigmentation**. The presence of scarring is a significant feature of invasive melanoma, with a specificity of 93% and a sensitivity of 36% (Figures 2.122–2.123).[4]

A specific form of depigmentation is the **white scar-like patch**. This is seen as a white stellate area normally found in a central position in more than half of dermatofibromas (Figure 2.126).[50] While much less common, white scar-like patches have been described in melanoma.[13,51] A variant of the white scar-like patch is the **white network**. It too is usually central in position and found in 18% of dermatofibromas.[50] The cords of the white network are usually thicker than the negative pigment network seen in some melanocytic lesions, however sometimes the morphology can be similar (Figure 2.84).

Follicular plugs and asymmetric pigmented follicular openings

Follicular plugs are seen as well-defined round "target" structures. Surprisingly, follicular plugs are a significant feature of invasive melanoma (Figures 2.127–2.129).[4] **Asymmetric pigmented follicular openings** refer to dark pigmentation in an asymmetric distribution around follicular openings. They are formed by an asymmetric descent of melanoma cells within individual hair follicles. They are seen in 68% of lentigo maligna but only 12% of benign pigmented macules of the face (Figures 2.130–2.131).[24]

Peripheral light-brown structureless areas

Peripheral light-brown structureless areas are seen as light-brown, variable-sized and shaped areas found at the periphery of a lesion and occupying more than 10% of its surface. This feature has a sensitivity of 63% and specificity of 96% for the diagnosis of thin melanoma[48] and a 19% sensitivity and 93% specificity for the diagnosis of hypomelanotic melanoma.[13] Histologically the areas are due to relative flattening of the rete ridges in combination with a preponderance of single cell pagetoid melanoma cells and pigmented keratinocytes rather than the formation of nests in the epidermis (Figures 2.141–2.144).[48]

References

1. Bahmer, F, Fritsch, P, Kreusch, J, et al. Terminology in surface microscopy. *J Am Acad Dermatol* 1990; 23: 1159–62.

2. Soyer, H, Argenziano, G, Chimenti, S, Menzies, S, Pehamberger, H, Rabinovitz, H, Stolz, W, Kopf, A. *Dermoscopy of Pigmented Skin Lesions*. Milan, Italy: Edra: 2001.

3. Argenziano, G, Soyer, HP, Chimenti, S, et al. Dermoscopy of pigmented skin lesions: results of a consensus meeting via the Internet. *J Am Acad Dermatol* 2003; 48: 679-93.

4. Menzies, S, Ingvar, C, McCarthy, W. A sensitivity and specificity analysis of the surface microscopy features of invasive melanoma. *Melanoma Res* 1996; 6: 55–62.

5. Nachbar, F, Stolz, W, Merkle, T, et al. The ABCD rule of dermatoscopy. *J Am Acad Dermatol* 1994; 30: 551–9.

6. Nilles, M, Boedeker, R, Schill, W. Surface microscopy of naevi and melanomas—clues to melanoma. *Br J Dermatol* 1994; 130: 349–55.

7. Menzies, S, Ingvar, C, Crotty, K, McCarthy, W. Frequency and morphologic characteristics of invasive melanomas lacking specific surface microscopic features. *Arch Dermatol* 1996; 132: 1178–82.

8. Arevalo, A, Altamura, D, Avramidis, M, Blum, A, Menzies, SW. The significance of eccentric and central hyperpigmentation, multifocal hyper-hypopigmentation and the multicomponent pattern in melanocytic lesions lacking specific dermoscopy features of melanoma. *Arch Dermatol* 2008; 144: 1440–4.

9. Yadav, S, Vossaert, KA, Kopf, AW, Silverman, M, Grin-Jorgensen, C. Histopathologic correlates of structures seen on dermoscopy (epiluminescence microscopy). *Am J Dermatopathol* 1993; 15: 297–305.

10. Kenet, R, Kang, S, Kenet, B, et al. Clinical diagnosis of pigmented lesions using digital epiluminescence microscopy. *Arch Dermatol* 1993; 129: 157–74.

11. Pehamberger, H, Binder, M, Steiner, A, Wolff, K. In vivo epiluminescence microscopy: Improvement of early diagnosis of melanoma. *J Invest Dermatol* 1993; 100: 356S–62S.

12. Massi, D, De Giorgi, V, Carli, P, Santucci, M. Diagnostic significance of the blue hue in dermoscopy of melanocytic lesions: a dermoscopic-pathologic study. *Am J Dermatopathol* 2001; 23: 463–9.

13. Menzies, SW, Kreusch, J, Byth, K, Pizzichetta, MD, et al. Dermoscopy of amelanotic and hypomelanotic melanoma. *Arch Dermatol* 2008; 144: 1120–7.

14. Soyer, H, Smolle, J, Hodl, S, et al. Surface Microscopy. A new approach to the diagnosis of cutaneous pigmented tumors. *Am J Dermatopath* 1989; 11: 1–10.

15. Rezze, GG, Scramim, AP, Neves, RI, Landman, G. Structural correlations between dermoscopic features of cutaneous melanomas and histopathology using transverse sections. *Am J Dermatopathol* 2006; 28: 13–20.

16. Steiner, A, Binder, M, Schemper, M, et al. Statistical evaluation of epiluminescence microscopy criteria for melanocytic pigment skin lesions. *J Am Acad Dermatol* 1993; 29: 581–8.

17. Puppin, D, Salomon, D, Saurat, J. Amplified surface microscopy. *J Am Acad Dermatol* 1993; 28: 923–7.

18. Menzies, S, Crotty, K, McCarthy, W. The morphologic criteria of the pseudopod in surface microscopy. *Arch Dermatol* 1995; 131: 436–40.

19. Steiner, A, Pehamberger, H, Binder, M, Wolff, K. Pigmented Spitz nevi: Improvement of the diagnostic accuracy by epiluminescence microscopy. *J Am Acad Dermatol* 1992; 27: 697–701.

20. Kreusch, J, Rassner, G. Strukturanalyse melanozytischer pigmentmale durch auflichtmikroskopie. *Hautarzt* 1990; 41: 27–33.

21. Barnhill, R, Mihm, M. The histopathology of cutaneous malignant melanoma. *Seminars in Diagnostic Pathology* 1993; 10(1): 47–75.

22. Fritsch, P, Pechlaner, R. The pigmented network: A new tool for the diagnosis of pigmented lesions. *J Invest Dermatol* 1980; 74: 458–9.

23. Zalaudek, I, Argenziano, G, Ferrara, G, et al. Clinically equivocal melanocytic skin lesions with features of regression: a dermoscopic-pathological study. *Br J Dermatol* 2004; 150(1): 64–71.

24. Schiffner, R, Schiffner-Rohe, J, Vogt, T, Landthaler, M, Wlotzke, U, Cognetta, A, Stolz, W. Improvement of early recognition of lentigo maligna using dermatoscopy. *J Am Acad Dermatol* 2000; 42: 25–32.

25. Braun, RP, Gaide, O, Oliviero, M, Kopf, AW, French, LE, Saurat, JH, Rabinovitz, HS. The significance of multiple blue-grey dots (granularity) for the dermoscopic diagnosis of melanoma. *Br J Dermatol* 2007; 157: 907–13.

26. Demirtaşoglu, M, Ilknur, T, Lebe, B, Kuşku, E, Akarsu, S, Ozkan, S. Evaluation of dermoscopic and histopathologic features and their correlations in pigmented basal cell carcinomas. *J Eur Acad Dermatol Venereol* 2006; 20: 916–20.

27. Changchien, L, Dusza, SW, Agero, AL, Korzenko, AJ, Braun, RP, Sachs, D, Usman, MH, Halpern, AC, Marghoob, AA. Age- and site-specific variation in

the dermoscopic patterns of congenital melanocytic nevi: an aid to accurate classification and assessment of melanocytic nevi. *Arch Dermatol* 2007; 143: 1007–14.

28. Ingordo, V, Iannazzone, SS, Cusano, F, Naldi, L. Dermoscopic features of congenital melanocytic nevus and Becker nevus in an adult male population: an analysis with a 10-fold magnification. *Dermatol* 2006; 212(4): 354–60.

29. Seidenari, S, Pellacani, G, Martella, A, Giusti, F. Instrument-, age- and site-dependent variations of dermoscopic patterns of congenital melanocytic naevi: a multicentre study. *Br J Dermatol* 2006; 155: 56–61

30. Saida, T, Koga, H. Dermoscopic patterns of acral melanocytic nevi: their variations, changes, and significance. *Arch Dermatol* 2007; 143: 1423–6

31. Miyazaki, A, Saida, T, Koga, H, Oguchi, S, Suzuki, T, Tsuchida, T. Anatomical and histopathological correlates of the dermoscopic patterns seen in melanocytic nevi on the sole: a retrospective study. *J Am Acad Dermatol* 2005; 53: 230–6.

32. Kimoto, M, Sakamoto, M, Iyatomi, H, Tanaka, M. Three-dimensional melanin distribution of acral melanocytic nevi is reflected in dermoscopy features: analysis of the parallel pattern. *Dermatology* 2008; 216: 205–12.

33. Palleschi, GM, Cipollini, EM, Torchia, D, Torre, E, Urso, C. Fibrillar pattern of a plantar acquired melanocytic naevus: correspondence between epiluminescence microscopy and transverse section histology. *Clin Exp Dermatol* 2006; 31: 449–51.

34. Saida, T, Miyazaki, A, Oguchi, S, Ishihara, Y, Yamazaki, Y, Murase, S, Yoshikawa, S, Tsuchida, T, Kawabata, Y, Tamaki, K. Significance of dermoscopic patterns in detecting malignant melanoma on acral volar skin: results of a multicenter study in Japan. *Arch Dermatol* 2004; 140: 1233–8.

35. Steiner, A, Pehamberger, H, Binder, M, Wolff, K. Pigmented Spitz nevi: Improvement of the diagnostic accuracy by epiluminescence microscopy. *J Am Acad Dermatol* 1992; 27: 697–701.

36. Menzies, S, Westerhoff, K, Rabinovitz, H, Kopf, A, McCarthy, W, Katz, B. The surface microscopy of pigmented basal cell carcinoma. *Arch Dermatol* 2000; 136: 1012–16.

37. Argenziano, G, Zalaudek, I, Corona R, et al. Vascular structures in skin tumors: a dermoscopy study. *Arch Dermatol* 2004; 140: 1485–9.

38. Zaballos, P, Daufi, C, Puig, S, Argenziano, G, Moreno-Ramírez, D, Cabo, H, Marghoob, AA, Llambrich, A, Zalaudek, I, Malvehy, J. Dermoscopy of solitary angiokeratomas: a morphological study. *Arch Dermatol* 2007; 143: 318–25.

39. Pizzichetta, MA, Talamini, R, Stanganelli, I, et al. Amelanotic/hypomelanotic melanoma: clinical and dermoscopic features. *Br J Dermatol* 2004; 150: 1117–24.

40. Stolz, W, Braun-Falco, O, Bilek, P, Landthaler, M, Cognetta, A (eds). *Color Atlas of Dermatoscopy*, 1st edn. Blackwell Science, Oxford, 1994.

41. Bono, R, Giampetruzzi, AR, Concolino, F, Puddu, P, Scoppola, A, Sera, F, Marchetti, P. Dermoscopic patterns of cutaneous melanoma metastases. *Melanoma Res* 2004; 14: 367–73.

42. Zalaudek, I, Argenziano, G, Leinweber, B, Citarella, L, Hofmann-Wellenhof, R, Malvehy, J, Puig, S, Pizzichetta, MA, Thomas L, Soyer HP, Kerl H. Dermoscopy of Bowen's disease. *Br J Dermatol* 2004; 150: 1112–6.

43. Vázquez-López, F, Zaballos, P, Fueyo-Casado, A, Sánchez-Martín, J. A dermoscopy subpattern of plaque-type psoriasis: red globular rings. *Arch Dermatol* 2007; 143: 1612.

44. Bugatti, L, Filosa, G, Broganelli, P, Tomasini, C. Psoriasis-like dermoscopic pattern of clear cell acanthoma. *J Eur Acad Dermatol Venereol* 2003; 17: 452–5.

45. Zalaudek, I, Hofmann-Wellenhof, R, Argenziano, G. Dermoscopy of clear-cell acanthoma differs from dermoscopy of psoriasis. *Dermatology* 2003; 207: 428.

46. Vázquez-López, F, Zaballos, P, Fueyo-Casado, A, Sánchez-Martín, J. A dermoscopy subpattern of plaque-type psoriasis: red globular rings. *Arch Dermatol* 2007; 143: 1612.

47. Blum, A, Metzler, G, Bauer, J, Rassner, G, Garbe, C. The dermatoscopic pattern of clear-cell acanthoma resembles psoriasis vulgaris. *Dermatology* 2001; 203: 50–2.

48. Annessi, G, Bono, R, Sampogna, F, Faraggiana, T, Abeni, D. Sensitivity, specificity, and diagnostic accuracy of three dermoscopic algorithmic methods

in the diagnosis of doubtful melanocytic lesions: the importance of light brown structureless areas in differentiating atypical melanocytic nevi from thin melanomas. *J Am Acad Dermatol* 2007; 56: 759–67.

49. Kopf, AW, Rabinovitz, H, Marghoob, A, Braun, RP, Wang, S, Oliviero, M, Polsky, D. "Fat fingers:" a clue in the dermoscopic diagnosis of seborrheic keratoses. *J Am Acad Dermatol* 2006; 55: 1089–91.

50. Zaballos, P, Puig, S, Llambrich, A, Malvehy, J. Dermoscopy of dermatofibromas: a prospective morphological study of 412 cases. *Arch Dermatol* 2008; 144: 75–83.

51. Blum, A, Bauer, J. Atypical dermatofibroma-like pattern of a melanoma on dermoscopy. *Melanoma Res* 2003; 13: 633–4.

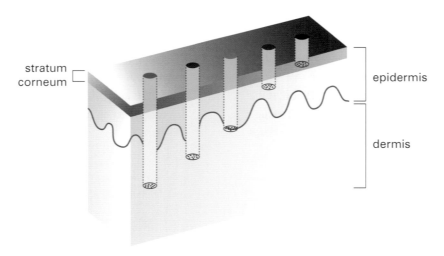

FIGURE 2.1 Melanin pigmentation

The color of melanin as seen under surface microscopy depends upon its histological level and density. In small quantities (e.g. in single cells or small groups of melanin-containing cells) melanin is seen as black when found within the stratum corneum, dark brown within the epidermis, tan at or near the dermoepidermal junction, gray in the upper dermis and blue in the mid to lower dermis. When present in large quantities, epidermal melanin can appear as black, even though the stratum corneum may lack any pigment (e.g. in some examples of lentigo simplex).

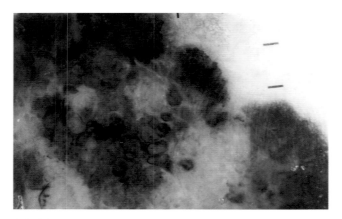

FIGURE 2.2 Multiple colors

The presence of 5 or 6 colors (tan, dark brown, black, gray, red and blue) has a specificity of 92% and a sensitivity of 53% for invasive melanoma. All six colors are present in this superficial spreading melanoma. The measurement gradations shown are 2 mm.

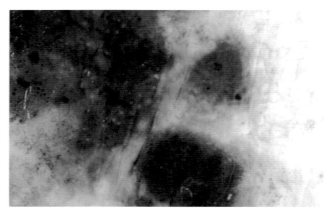

FIGURE 2.3 Multiple colors in an invasive melanoma

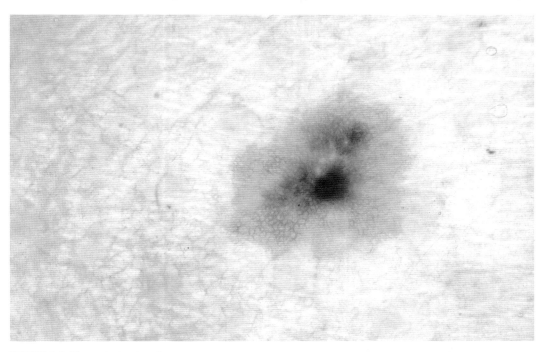

FIGURE 2.4 Pigmented network

The pigmented network is the unifying surface microscopic feature of melanocytic-derived lesions and is found in many examples of the lentigo, lentiginous, junctional and compound nevus (common and dysplastic), and melanoma. This lesion is a lentigo.

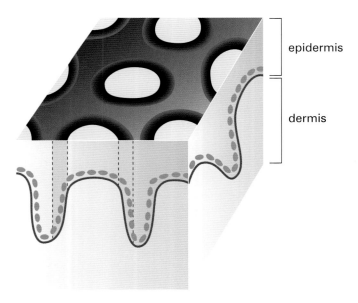

epidermis

dermis

FIGURE 2.5 Pigmented network—histopathology*

The pigmented network is formed by melanocytes, pigmented keratinocytes or melanocyte-derived cells at the basal layer of the epidermis. When viewed vertically with the surface microscope, these cells produce areas of dense pigment due to projections of the rete pegs/ridges (constituting the grids of the network) and relatively little pigment due to the projections of the dermal papillae (constituting the holes of the network).

This figure is derived from: Fritsch, P, Pechlaner, R. Differentiation of benign from malignant melanocytic lesions using incident light microscopy. In: Ackerman A (ed.). Pathology of malignant melanoma, New York, Masson, 1981; pp. 301–12.

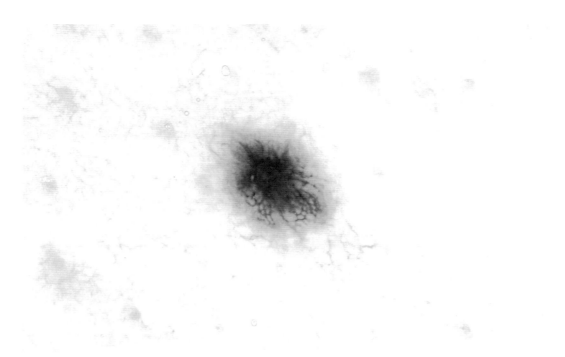

FIGURE 2.6 Pigment network (wide)
The anatomical site influences the pattern of the network by determining the pattern of the rete ridges. In this dysplastic compound nevus the network "holes" have a wide diameter.

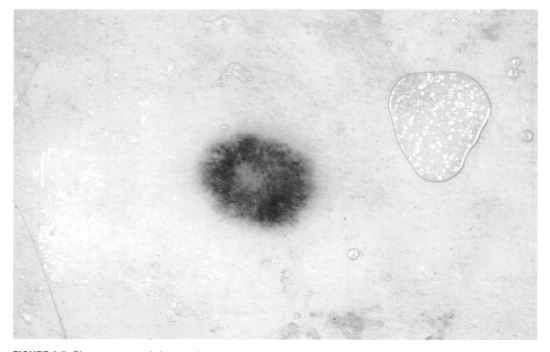

FIGURE 2.7 Pigment network (narrow)
In this compound nevus the network "holes" have a narrow diameter.

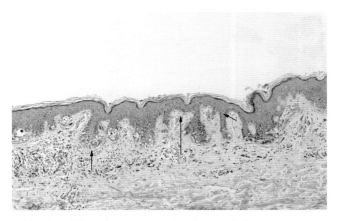

FIGURE 2.8 Wide pigment network—histopathology
In this melanocytic nevus the pigmented rete ridges (medium arrow) form the "grids" of the network and the wide diameter dermal papillae (large arrow) form the "holes" of the network. Note that the majority of pigment is found in basal keratinocytes (small arrow) and melanocytes rather than the nevus cells. Magnification ×25 (H & E stain).

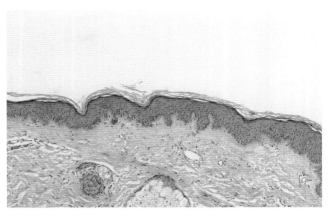

FIGURE 2.10 Diffuse pigmentation—histopathology
When the rete ridges are poorly defined (relatively flat) as seen in this lentigo, no pigment network is seen. Instead, these lesions are seen under dermoscopy as areas of diffuse brown pigmentation (see Figure 2.22). Note that diffuse brown pigmentation can also be seen in lesions with pigmented cells high in the papillary dermis near the dermoepidermal junction. Magnification ×25 (H & E stain).

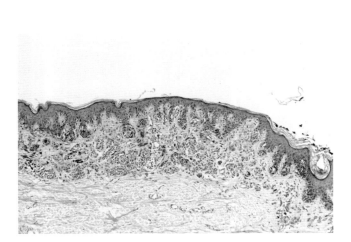

FIGURE 2.9 Narrow pigment network—histopathology
In this melanocytic nevus the dermal papillae are narrow in width leaving a relatively narrow distance between the pigmented rete ridges. This results in a narrow pigment network. Magnification ×25 (H & E stain).

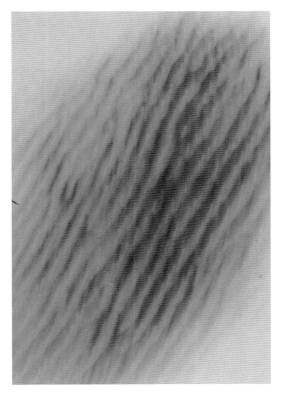

FIGURE 2.11 Pigment network volar—Parallel furrow/pattern
The pigment network on volar sites (palms and soles) has a different morphological appearance to the network seen elsewhere. The most common pattern seen in benign volar nevi is the parallel furrow pattern, where the thin parallel furrows of the surface skin markings are preferentially pigmented and the broader ridges are hypopigmented. This pattern is preferentially seen on the non-arch surface of the sole of the foot.

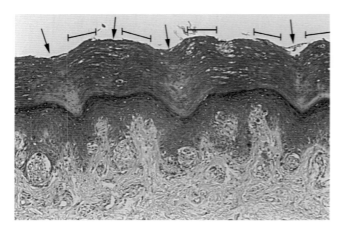

FIGURE 2.12 Parallel furrow pattern—histopathology

The keratin layer (stratum corneum) in acral skin is thick and there are obvious ridges (space bars) and furrows (arrows) which correspond to the skin markings or fingerprints. In this predominantly junctional acral naevus the pigment in the stratum corneum is concentrated in the *furrows*. The nests of junctional melanocytes are concentrated at the tips of the rete ridges beneath these furrows (the crista profunda limitans). Melanin is therefore found in a column from the crista profunda limitans up to and including the stratum corneum. This vertical column of melanin gives the dermoscopy appearance of the parallel furrows of the skin surface markings being preferentially pigmented. Magnification ×50 (H & E stain).

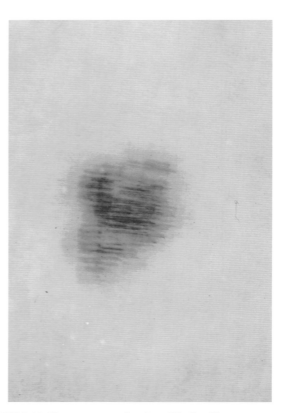

FIGURE 2.14 Pigment network volar—Fibrillar/filamentous pattern

This nevus on the sole of foot has the fibrillar/filamentous pattern. Here a mesh-like or delicate filamentous pigmentation crossing the lines of skin markings is seen. This pattern is seen in nevi on the weight bearing surface of the foot and is due to the column of melanin found in the parallel furrow pattern seen in a slanting rather than vertical position.

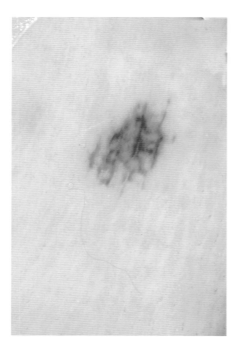

FIGURE 2.13 Pigment network volar–Parallel furrow/lattice pattern

Here the parallel furrow pattern is preserved but additionally has lines crossing the furrows forming a lattice pattern. This pattern is seen in nevi on the arch of the foot.

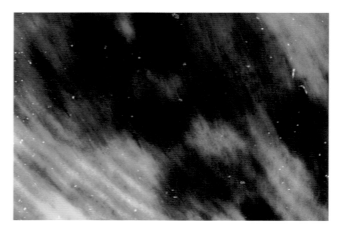

FIGURE 2.15 Pigment network volar—Parallel ridge pattern

On volar sites the parallel ridge pattern has a sensitivity of 86% and specifically of 99% for the diagnosis of melanoma (both invasive and in situ). Here the ridges of the surface skin markings (in contrast to the narrow furrows as in Figure 2.11) are predominantly pigmented. Hence the width of the pigmented lines are greater in the parallel ridge pattern in comparison with the parallel furrow/lattice-like patterns.

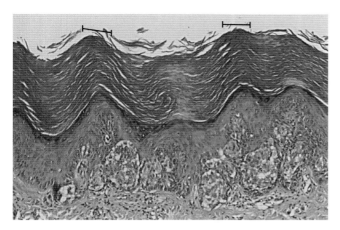

FIGURE 2.16 Parallel ridge pattern—histopathology

In this acral lentiginous melanoma there are confluent nests of atypical melanocytes involving the basal and mid epidermis. The pigment is concentrated in the ridges of the keratin layer (delineated by space bars). Beneath these pigmented ridges the atypical melanocytes are more concentrated. Magnification ×50 (H & E stain).

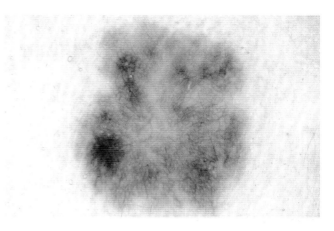

FIGURE 2.17 Pigment network—discrete regular

A discrete (lightly pigmented) network that also has a regular width of the grids (cords) making up the net (discrete/regular network) is generally found in benign melanocytic lesions such as the ephelis, solar lentigo, and junctional and compound nevus (as in Figure 2.4). A discrete/regular network is found in only 7% of melanomas and is a significant negative correlate of melanoma. In this predominantly junctional nevus, the discrete regular network is seen to blend into normal skin at the edge of the lesion. This **graduated network edge** is a feature of benign melanocytic lesions. In contrast, an **abrupt network edge** is a common feature of dysplastic nevi and melanoma (see Figure 2.19 and Figure 2.20). Finally, a discrete regular network is also commonly found in dermatofibromas (see Figure 2.126)

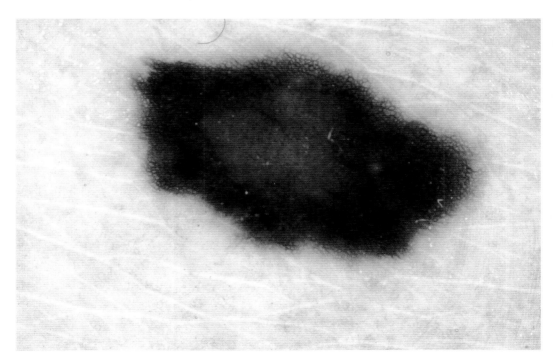

FIGURE 2.18 Pigment network—prominent irregular

A prominent (darkly pigmented) network with irregular-width grids (**prominent/irregular network**) is often found in dysplastic nevi, and in in situ and invasive melanoma. However, using the low power magnification of the hand-held surface microscope, a prominent/irregular network is not a statistically significant feature of invasive melanoma. This figure shows a prominent/irregular network in a dysplastic nevus.

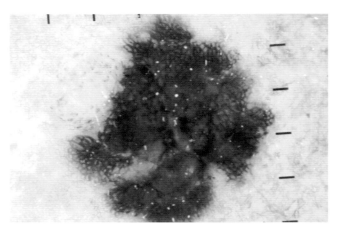

FIGURE 2.19 Pigment network—broadened

A network with broad width cords (broadened network) is a significant finding of melanoma. While it is the commonest feature of lentigo maligna (Hutchinson's melanotic freckle), it also has specificity for invasive melanoma (specificity 86% and sensitivity 35%). This is a superficial spreading melanoma. Note the abrupt network edge at the skin–lesion border, a significant finding in invasive melanoma.

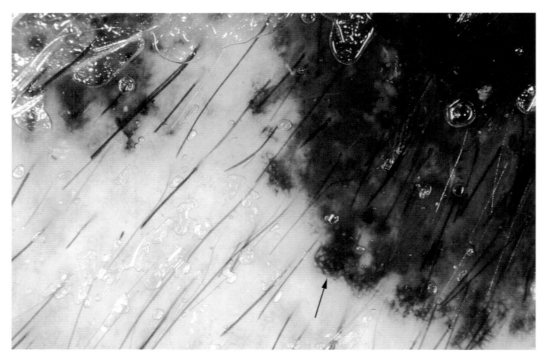

FIGURE 2.20 Pigment network—broadened

Areas of prominent broadened network (arrow) are seen at the edge of this superficial spreading melanoma. Broadened network is usually found focally rather than throughout a lesion.

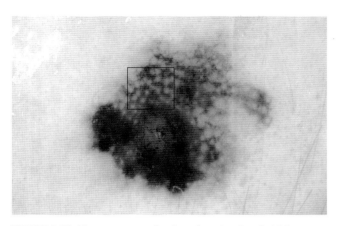

FIGURE 2.21 Pigment network—broadened—rhomboidal structures
The broadened network of lentigo maligna or lentigo maligna melanoma on the face can form dark (brown to black) rhomboidal structures (seen within the box). These occur in 49% of lentigo maligna but are absent in the majority of benign pigmented macules of the face.

FIGURE 2.23 Pigment network—pseudo-broadened
The dilated follicular openings seen on the face often create a uniform false broadened network in benign pigmented macules, such as the ephelis, lentigo, actinic keratosis and junctional nevus. This is a facial solar lentigo.

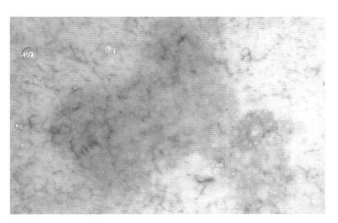

FIGURE 2.22 Uniform pigment pattern (diffuse pigmentation)
The solitary finding of a uniform diffuse background of *brown* pigmentation occurs in most examples of the ephelis (freckle), and in some examples of the actinic (solar) lentigo and compound nevus. This lesion is a solar lentigo. This feature should be contrasted with peripheral light brown stuctureless areas found in melanoma (Figures 2.141–2.144) since this latter feature occurs only in a peripheral position of the lesion.

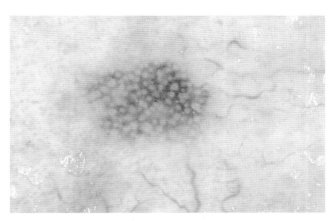

FIGURE 2.24 Pseudo-broadened pigment network in a junctional nevus on the face

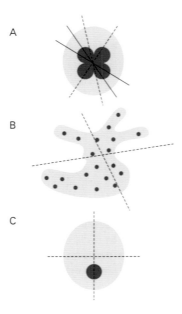

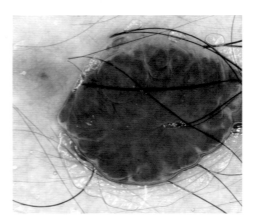

FIGURE 2.27 Symmetrical pigmentation pattern in a dermal nevus

FIGURE 2.25 Pattern symmetry definitions
A. **Symmetrical pigmentation pattern** refers to symmetry of pattern/ texture over *all* axes through the center (of gravity) of a lesion. It does *not* require symmetry of shape. Here, the schematic lesion has mirror symmetry across any axis through its center—hence it has a symmetrical pigmentation pattern. B. Here, while the lesion lacks symmetry of shape, its repeated pattern results in symmetrical pigmentation pattern. C. While this lesion has symmetry of pattern over its long axis, it lacks symmetry over its short axis. Hence the lesion has an **asymmetric pigmentation pattern**.

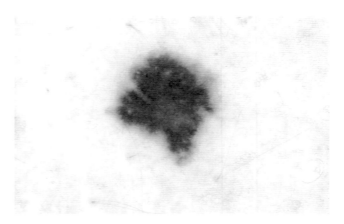

FIGURE 2.28 Symmetrical pigmentation pattern in a dysplastic nevus
Note that the symmetry in symmetrical pigmentation pattern refers to the pigmentation pattern and *not* the shape.

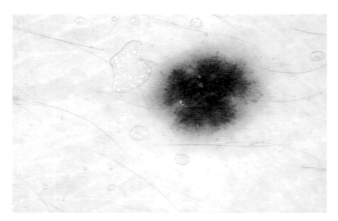

FIGURE 2.26 Symmetrical pigmentation pattern
Clear, precise symmetry never occurs in biological tissue but rather approximates the situation. This lesion has symmetry of pattern over all axes through its centre. The presence of symmetrical pigmentation pattern is often the defining feature of benign pigmented lesions.

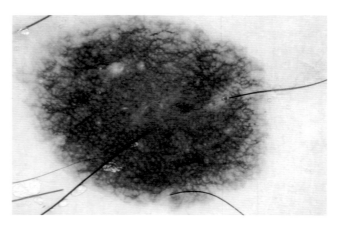

FIGURE 2.29 Symmetrical pigmentation pattern in a dysplastic nevus

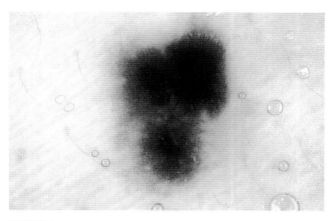

FIGURE 2.30 Asymmetric pigmentation pattern

Asymmetric pigmentation pattern is found in lesions that lack symmetry over one or more axes through its center. This feature has a specificity of 46% and a sensitivity approaching 100% for invasive melanoma (i.e. nearly all invasive melanoma have asymmetric pigmentation, but 54% of atypical non-melanoma pigmented lesions also have this feature). This lesion is a dysplastic junctional nevus.

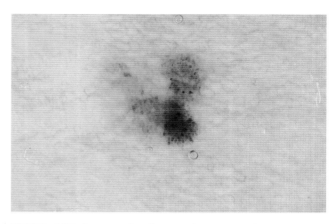

FIGURE 2.33 Asymmetric pigmentation pattern in an invasive melanoma

FIGURE 2.31 Asymmetric pigmentation pattern in a dysplastic nevus

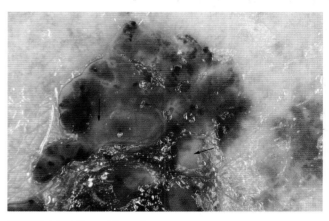

FIGURE 2.34 Blue-white veil

Blue-white veil (arrows) is seen as an irregular area of indistinct, structureless, confluent blue pigment with an overlying white ground-glass film. It cannot be associated with red-blue areas (lacunes) (Figure 2.40). It is the single most significant dermoscopic finding of invasive melanoma, with a sensitivity of 51% and a specificity of 97%. This lesion is an invasive melanoma.

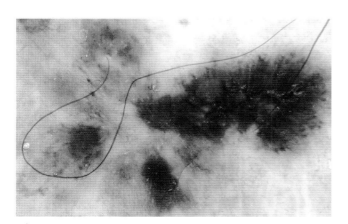

FIGURE 2.32 Asymmetric pigmentation pattern

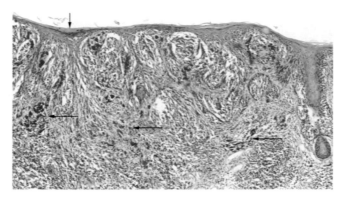

FIGURE 2.35 Blue-white veil—histopathology

Histopathologically the blue-white veil represents the presence of a compact aggregation of heavily pigmented cells (usually melanoma or melanophages) in the mid dermis (large arrow), in combination with thickened compact stratum corneum (compact orthokeratosis) (small arrow). The blue pigment is due to the mid-dermal melanin and the white veil (white ground-glass appearance) is due to the compact orthokeratosis. Magnification ×20 (H & E stain).

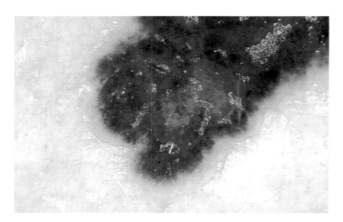

FIGURE 2.36 Blue-white veil in an invasive melanoma

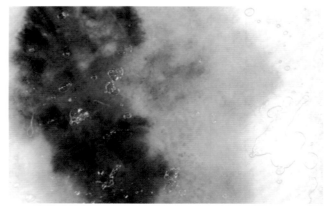

FIGURE 2.37 Blue-white veil in an invasive melanoma

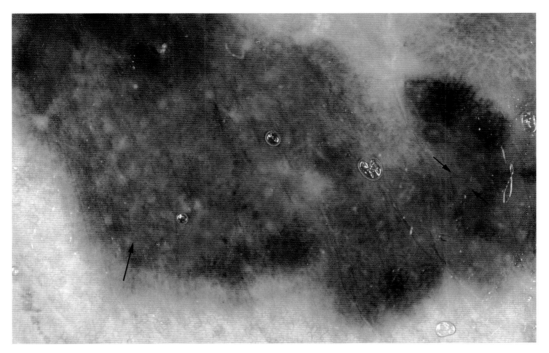

FIGURE 2.38 Blue-white veil in an invasive melanoma

The blue-white veil is seen as confluent blue pigment with a white overlying "ground-glass" film (delineated with small arrows). While it can be due to dense collections of melanophages, blue-white veil can be distinguished from multiple blue dots (large arrow) by the latter's lack of confluence of pigment.

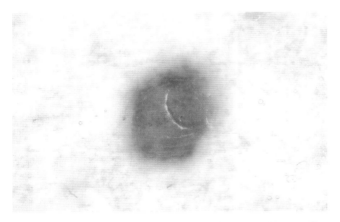

FIGURE 2.39 Differential diagnosis of blue-white veil— homogeneous blue pigmentation

Blue-white veil never occupies the entire surface area of the lesion and should be distinguished from the homogeneous blue pigmentation seen in most blue nevi. Many blue nevi (unlike the lesion seen here) also lack the white "ground-glass" film required to diagnose blue-white veil.

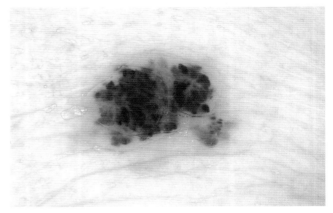

FIGURE 2.40 Differential diagnosis of blue-white veil

Blue-white veil cannot be associated with multiple red-blue areas (lacunes) seen in hemangiomas.

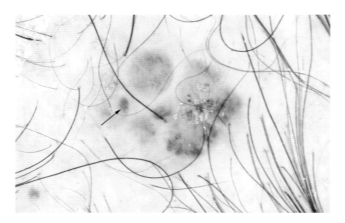

FIGURE 2.41 Differential diagnosis of blue-white veil
Blue-white veil is an indistinct and structureless feature. It should be distinguished from the discrete, ovoid nests (arrow) seen in pigmented basal cell carcinomas.

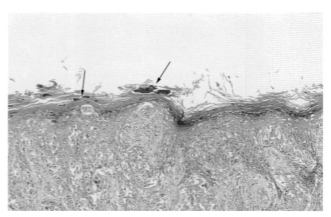

FIGURE 2.44 Black dots/globules—histopathology
Black dots/globules represent localized pigment accumulation (often melanoma cells) in the stratum corneum. The arrows show melanin in cells in the stratum corneum of an invasive melanoma. Magnification ×20 (H & E stain).

FIGURE 2.42 Differential diagnosis of blue-white veil
The central area of this compound nevus is not blue-white veil because it lacks the white veil and has discrete structure.

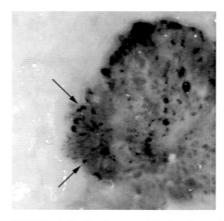

FIGURE 2.45 Black dots/globules (peripheral) in an invasive melanoma

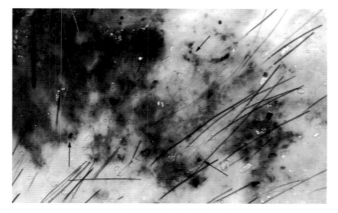

FIGURE 2.43 Black dots/globules (peripheral)
Black dots/globules found at or near the edge of a lesion (arrows) is a highly significant feature of invasive melanoma, with a specificity of 92% and a sensitivity of 42%. This lesion is an invasive melanoma.

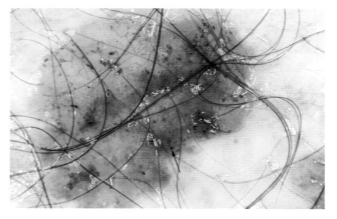

FIGURE 2.46 Black dots/globules (peripheral) in an invasive melanoma
The peripheral black dots present here (arrow), while being subtle, are enough to make the diagnosis of melanoma.

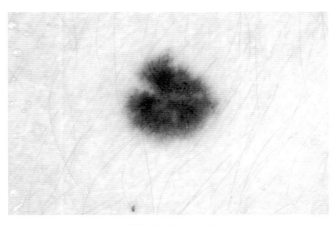

FIGURE 2.47 Black dots/globules (central)

Black dots/globules can be found in benign pigmented lesions, but tend to be relatively central in position. However, central black dots/globules are still a significant finding of invasive melanoma, with a specificity of 82% and a sensitivity of 51%. The figure shows central black dots/globules in a dysplastic nevus.

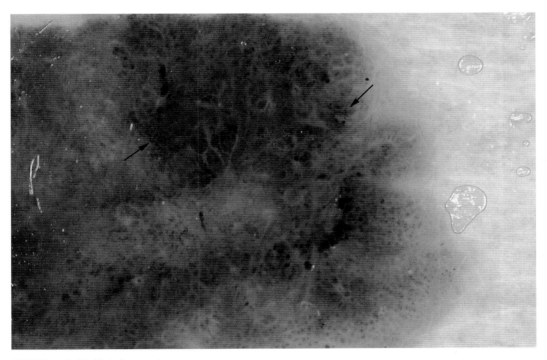

FIGURE 2.48 Multiple brown dots

Multiple brown dots are seen as focal aggregations of well-defined dark brown dots (delineated by arrows). This feature should be distinguished from that of scattered or isolated brown dots seen in many pigmented lesions (Figure 2.51). Multiple brown dots are a highly significant feature of invasive melanoma, with a specificity of 97% and a sensitivity of 30%. The lesion is an invasive melanoma.

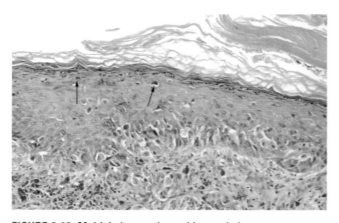

FIGURE 2.49 Multiple brown dots—histopathology

Multiple brown dots represent intraepidermal (supra-basal) pigment accumulation; usually single melanoma cells below the stratum corneum (arrows). Magnification ×50 (H & E stain).

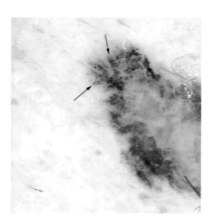

FIGURE 2.50 Multiple brown dots in an invasive melanoma

Note the focal nature of multiple brown dots.

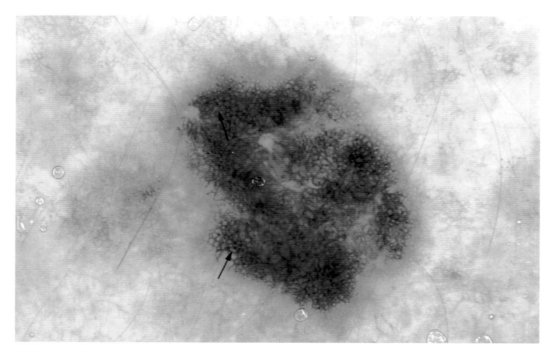

FIGURE 2.51 Brown dots/globules

Ovoid accumulation of brown pigment into scattered dots or globules is a common feature of many pigmented lesions, benign and malignant. In this junctional nevus the dots/globules are uniform in size and are mainly superimposed on the grids (cords) of the pigmented network (arrows). In dysplastic nevi and melanoma brown dots/globules tend to be irregular in shape and distribution.

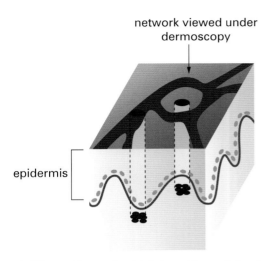

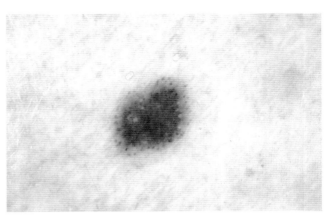

FIGURE 2.52 Brown dots/globules—histopathology†

Nests of pigmented cells at the tips of the rete pegs/ridges are seen under dermoscopy as brown globules superimposed on the grids of the network. Nests of pigmented cells in the dermal papilla are seen as brown globules in the "holes" of the network.

†This figure is derived from: Puppin, D, Salomon, D, Saurat, J. Amplified surface microscopy. J Am Acad Dermatol 1993; 28: 923–7.

FIGURE 2.54 Multiple peripheral brown globules

In one variant of dysplastic nevi, brown globules can be seen in a circumferential position defining the edge of the lesion. These are referred to as multiple peripheral brown globules. These nevi are often observed to have a rapid radial growth, but are benign.

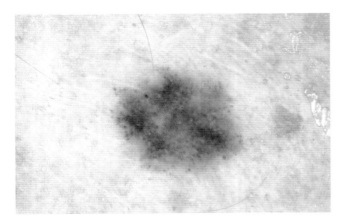

FIGURE 2.53 Brown dots/globules in a dysplastic nevus

Irregularly distributed brown globules with variable shapes and sizes are seen in this dysplastic nevus.

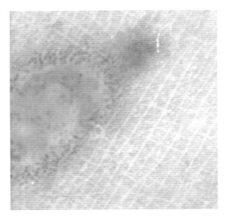

FIGURE 2.55 Multiple deep peripheral brown globules

In one variant of Spitz nevi, peripheral brown globules are seen in multiple layers.

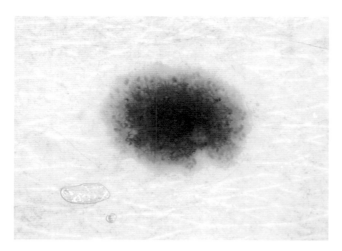

FIGURE 2.56 Aggregated globules

As in this lesion, significant proportions of compound nevi lack a pigment network. Areas of aggregated brown globules, seen here towards the periphery of the lesion, indicates the lesion is melanocytic in origin.

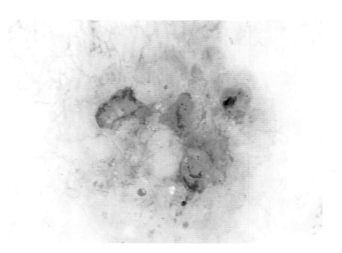

FIGURE 2.57 Ulceration

Ulceration occurs early in the evolution of basal cell carcinoma and late in invasive melanoma. It is found in 27% of pigmented BCC but only 13% of invasive melanoma and 1% of benign pigmented lesions. As in this case, when found in the absence of a pigmented network, it has a significant specificity for the diagnosis of pigmented BCC. For ulceration to be a significant feature there should not be a recent history of trauma.

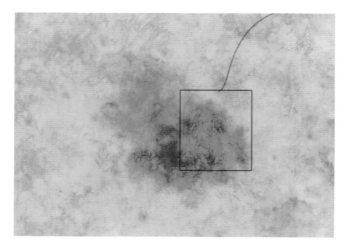

FIGURE 2.58 Fingerprint-like structures

Light brown fingerprint-like structures (delineated by the box) can be found in solar lentigo or early flat seborrheic keratoses. Fingerprint-like structures can be distinguished from a pigment network since the former has less net-like structures but rather has curvilinear thin brown cords.

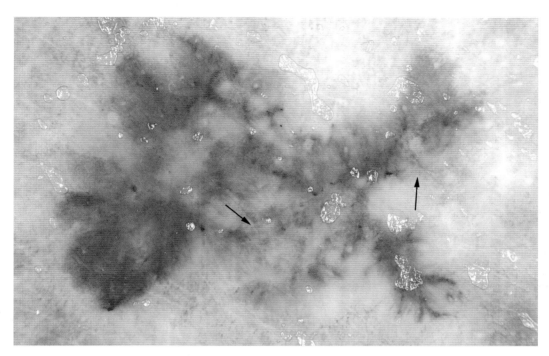

FIGURE 2.59 Multiple blue-gray dots (melanophages)

Multiple blue-gray dots are seen as diffuse, partly aggregated dots, often described as "pepper-like" in morphology. They are commonly seen in association with histological regression and therefore can be seen in any pigmented lesion. However, since regression is a common feature of malignant melanoma, the presence of multiple blue-gray dots is a significant feature of invasive melanoma, with a specificity of 91% and a sensitivity of 45%. This figure shows multiple blue dots (arrows) in a regressing superficial spreading melanoma. When focal multiple blue-gray dots are found in less than 10% of the surface area of a nevus lacking other specific dermoscopic features of melanoma (as seen in some dysplastic nevi), the lesion can be considered benign.

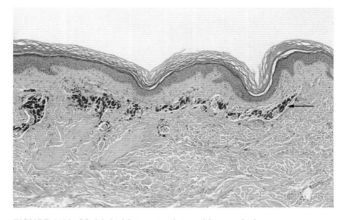

FIGURE 2.60 Multiple blue-gray dots—histopathology

Multiple blue-gray dots are melanophages in the dermis. Melanophages are melanin-laden macrophages that are particularly seen in regressed pigmented lesions. This section (of the lesion in Figure 2.62) shows multiple melanophages in the dermis. Magnification ×20 (H & E stain).

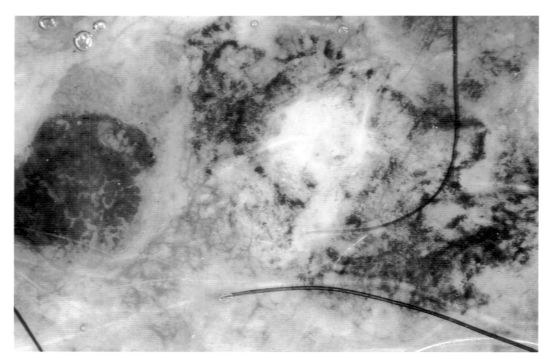

FIGURE 2.61 Multiple blue-gray dots in a lichen planus-like keratosis

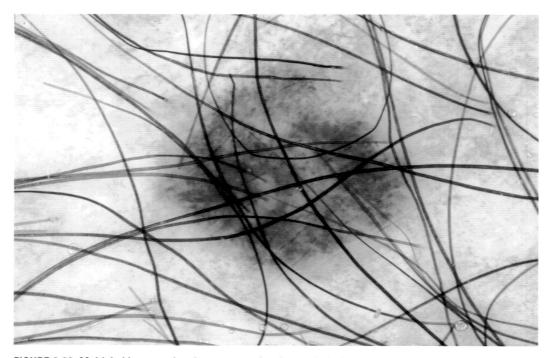

FIGURE 2.62 Multiple blue-gray dots in a regressed melanocytic lesion
When multiple melanophages become aggregated with a high density, they are seen as confluent areas of blue pigment.

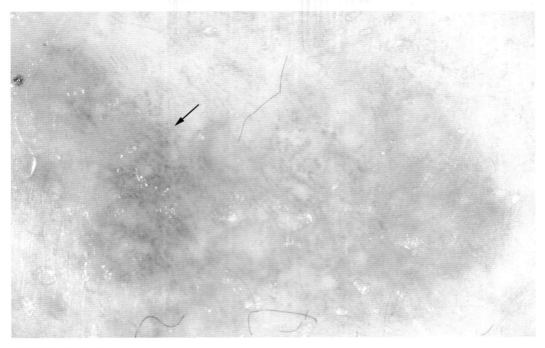

FIGURE 2.63 Multiple blue-gray dots in a regressing compound nevus
The color of melanophages depends on their depth in the dermis. These melanophages are seen as gray (arrow).

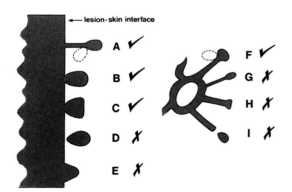

FIGURE 2.64 Pseudopods—morphological criteria‡
The pseudopod is one of the most morphologically variable features in dermoscopy. It is also one of the most specific features of superficial spreading melanoma, with a specificity of 97% and a sensitivity of 23%.

Because of the variability, a strict morphological definition is required. Pseudopods are bulbous and often kinked projections, which are directly connected to the tumor body (A, B, C) or pigmented network (F). When connected directly to the tumor body, they must have an acute angle to the tumor edge (B, C), or arise from linear or curvilinear extensions (A). When connected to the network (F), the width of the bulbous ending must be greater than the width of any part of the surrounding network (hence G is rejected) and at least double that of its directly connected network projection (hence H is rejected). Pseudopods cannot be diagnosed in the presence of multiple peripheral brown globules (Figure 2.54). The morphological forms satisfying the criteria are A, B, C and F; those that do not are D, E, G, H, and I.

‡This figure is from: Menzies, S, Crotty, K, McCarthy, W. The morphologic criteria of the pseudopod in surface microscopy. Arch Dermatol 1995; 131: 436–40.

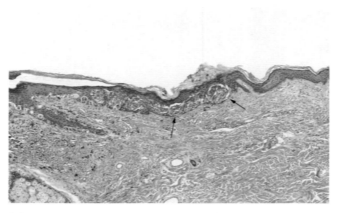

FIGURE 2.65 Pseudopods—histopathology[§]

Pseudopods represent junctional or intraepidermal radial nests of melanoma. In this section (from Figure 2.66), the pseudopod is cut through its long axis, and is seen as a radial intraepidermal nest of melanoma (arrows). Magnification ×20 (H & E stain).

[§]*This figure is from: Menzies, S. Crotty, K, McCarthy, W. The morphologic criteria of the pseudopod in surface microscopy.* Arch Dermatol *1995; 131: 436–40.*

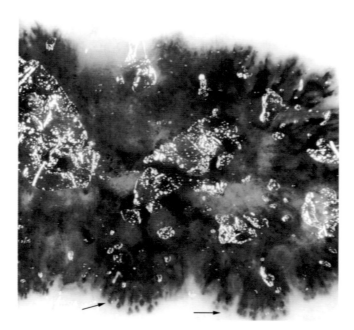

FIGURE 2.66 Pseudopods in a superficial spreading melanoma

Classical pseudopods are seen at the edge of this invasive melanoma (arrows).

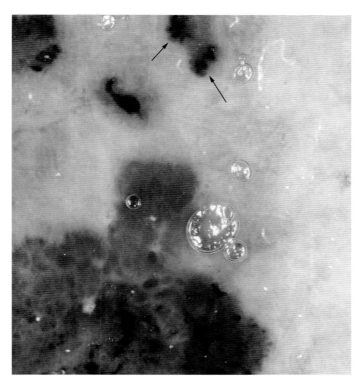

FIGURE 2.67 Pseudopods in a superficial spreading melanoma
Pseudopods (arrows) are heavily pigmented in 80% of cases.

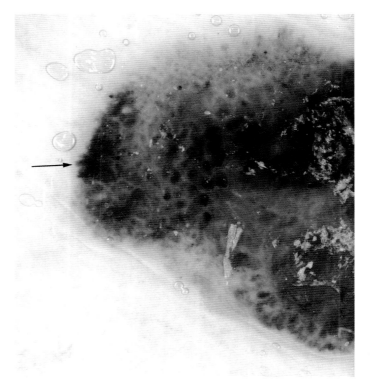

FIGURE 2.68 Pseudopods in a superficial spreading melanoma
These pseudopods arise directly from the tumor body.

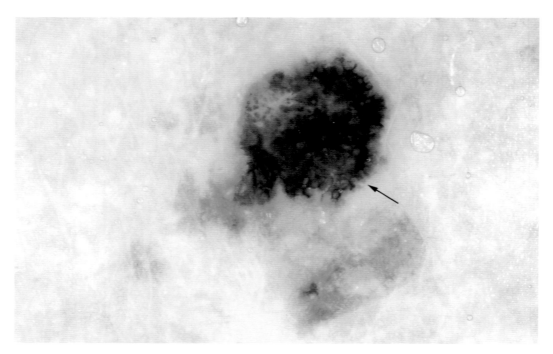

FIGURE 2.69 Pseudopods in a superficial spreading melanoma
These pseudopods arise from the pigment network.

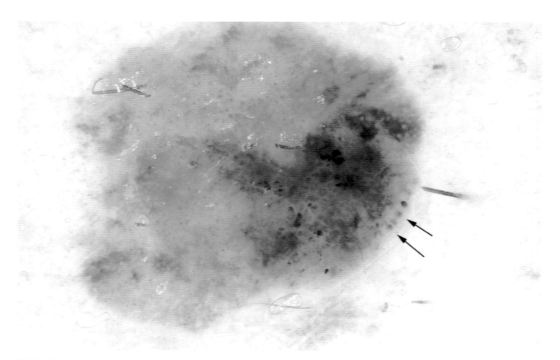

FIGURE 2.70 Pseudopods in a superficial spreading melanoma

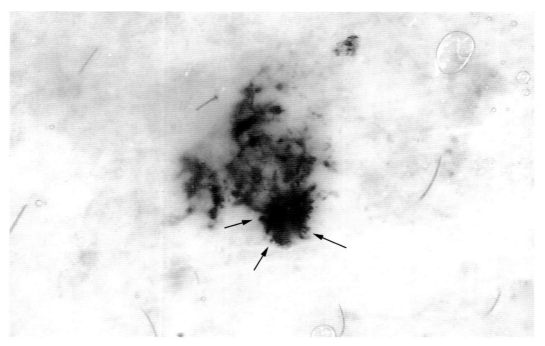

FIGURE 2.71 Pseudopods in a superficial spreading melanoma

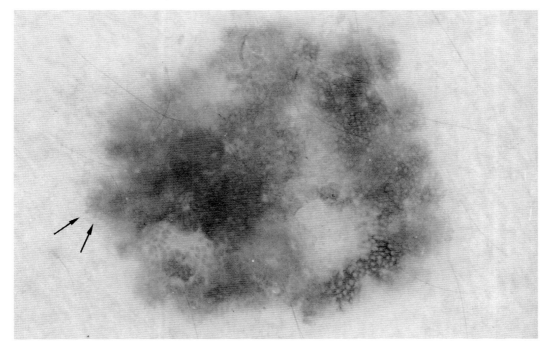

FIGURE 2.72 Pseudopods in a superficial spreading melanoma
The arrows show tan pseudopods in an early invasive melanoma. While these are subtle, they make the diagnosis of melanoma. This example illustrates the importance of carefully observing the edge of all pigmented lesions.

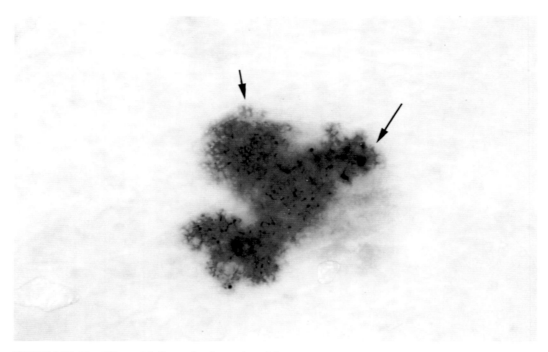

FIGURE 2.73 The differential diagnosis of pseudopods[¶]
Many structures resembling pseudopods are seen at the edge of the pigmented network in benign melanocytic nevi. The arrows indicate pseudopod-like structures in a dysplastic nevus that fails to meet the criteria defined in Figure 2.64 (rejected as in type G, large arrow; type H, small arrow).

[¶]*This figure is from: Menzies, S, Crotty, K, McCarthy, W. The morphologic criteria of the pseudopod in surface microscopy.* Arch Dermatol *1995; 131: 436–40.*

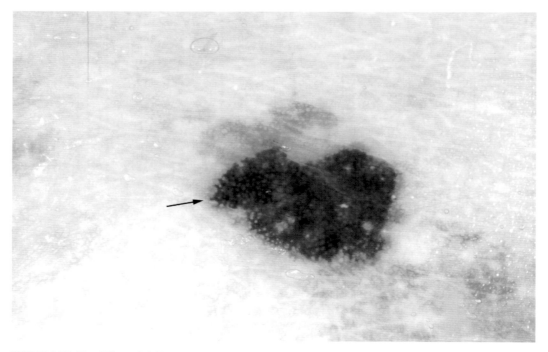

FIGURE 2.74 The differential diagnosis of pseudopods
The arrow indicates a pseudopod-like structure in a dysplastic nevus that is rejected as in type H (Figure 2.64).

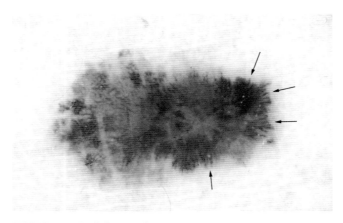

FIGURE 2.75 Radial streaming

Radial streaming is seen as radially and asymmetrically arranged parallel linear extensions at the edge of the tumor. Like the pseudopod, radial streaming represents histopathologically the radial growth phase of melanoma. While sometimes occurring within the body of a melanoma, radial streaming is a specific feature of melanoma only when seen at the edge. Under this definition, radial streaming has a specificity of 96% and a sensitivity of 18% for invasive melanoma. This lesion shows radial streaming in a superficial spreading melanoma (arrows).

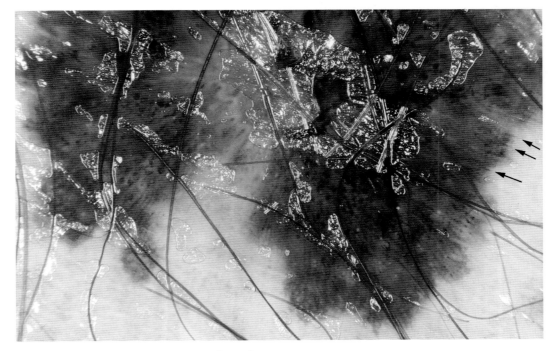

FIGURE 2.76 Radial streaming in an invasive melanoma

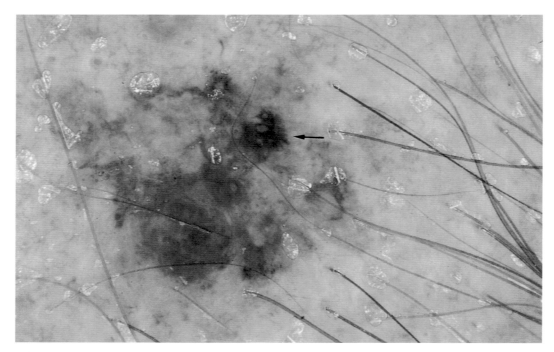

FIGURE 2.77 Radial streaming in an invasive melanoma

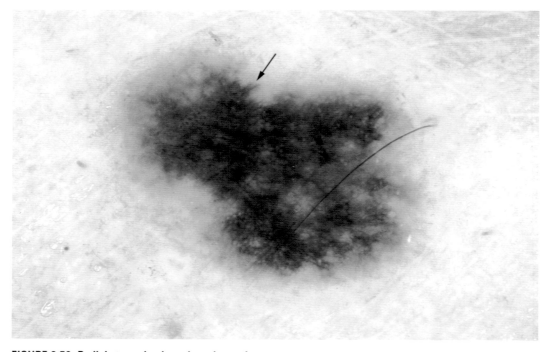

FIGURE 2.78 Radial streaming in an invasive melanoma
Radial streaming can be a very subtle feature. In this superficial spreading melanoma it is the only feature that distinguishes the lesion as malignant (arrow).

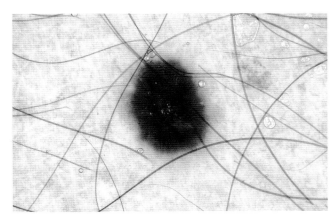

FIGURE 2.79 The differential diagnosis of radial streaming

Radial streaming should be seen at the edge of a lesion, rather than in the central position as in this dysplastic nevus. In addition, radial streaming is asymmetrical, unlike the circumferential regular distribution seen here. This lesion is a dysplastic compound nevus.

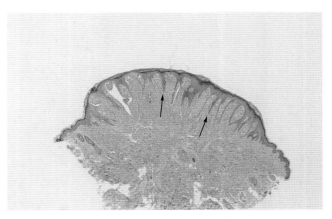

FIGURE 2.81 Negative pigment network—histopathology

Histopathologically the negative pigment network represents elongated hypomelanotic rete ridges (pegs) (arrows). This is a section from the Spitz nevus in Figure 2.80. Magnification ×5 (H & E stain).

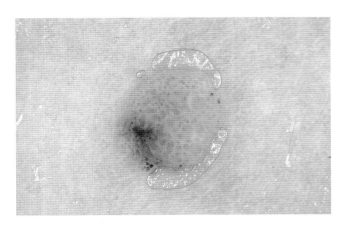

FIGURE 2.80 Negative pigment network

A negative pigment network is seen as a "negative" of the pigmented network, with light areas making up the grids of the network and dark areas filling the "holes". While it is seen commonly in Spitz nevi (as shown here), it is also a feature of invasive melanoma.

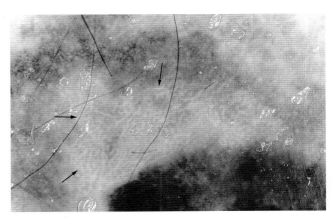

FIGURE 2.82 Negative pigment network in melanoma

The negative pigment network (in the area outlined by arrows) is a highly specific feature of invasive melanoma (95% specificity, 22% sensitivity). For this reason, the presence of a negative pigment network should not be used as an independent feature to diagnose Spitz nevi.

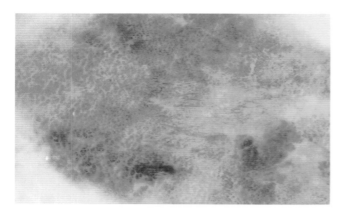

FIGURE 2.83 Negative pigment network in melanoma

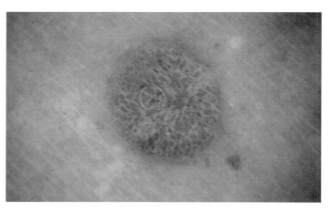

FIGURE 2.84 White network**

The cords of the white network are sometimes thicker than the negative pigment network seen in some melanocytic lesions, however sometimes the morphology can be indistinguishable (as seen here). It is usually central in position and found in 18% of dermatofibromas.

**This photograph was kindly provided by Dr Maria Pizzichetta, Italy.

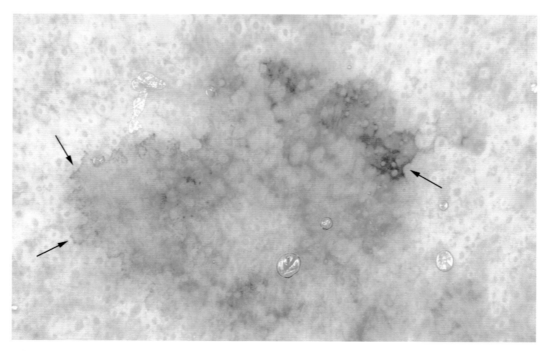

FIGURE 2.85 Moth-eaten edge

A moth-eaten edge is seen as well-defined "punched-out" concave areas at the edge of a lesion. While it is a common feature of the ephelis (freckle), it can also be seen occasionally in the lentigo, seborrheic keratosis and lentigo maligna.

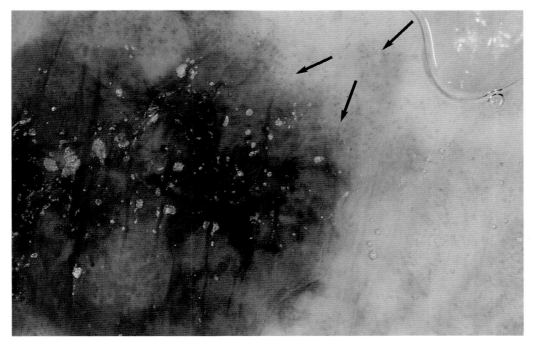

FIGURE 2.86 Telangiectases—dotted (pin point)

Telangiectases (dilated vessels in the papillary dermis) are more readily seen with dermoscopy. Care should be taken to avoid excessive pressure when examining vessel morphology. The use of ultrasound gel at the surface microscope-skin interface can reduce the need for pressure and therefore assist in examining vessels. Dotted vessels (arrows) are found in melanocytic tumors and occur in the same frequency in nevi and melanomas.

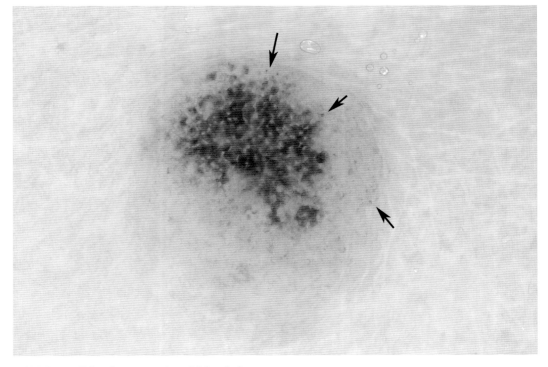

FIGURE 2.87 Telangiectases—dotted (pinpoint)

Here dotted vessels (arrows) are seen in this compound nevus.

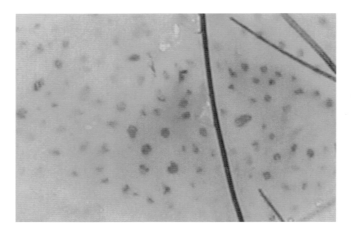

FIGURE 2.88 Telangiectases—glomerular (magnified image)
Larger dotted vessels giving the appearance of the capillaries of the renal glomerulus (glomerular vessels) are found in Bowen's disease, psoriatic plaques, and clear cell acanthomas. While this image is magnified, such morphology is easily seen with ×10 surface microscopes.

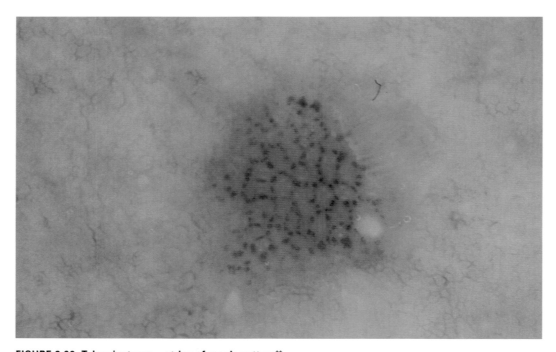

FIGURE 2.89 Telangiectases—string of pearls pattern[††]
Glomerular vessels seen as a reticular-linear "string of pearls" pattern occur most specifically in clear cell acanthomas (as seen here). However, a variant of this pattern can be seen in plaque psoriasis.

[††]This photograph was kindly provided by Dr Giuseppe Argenziano, Napoli, Italy.

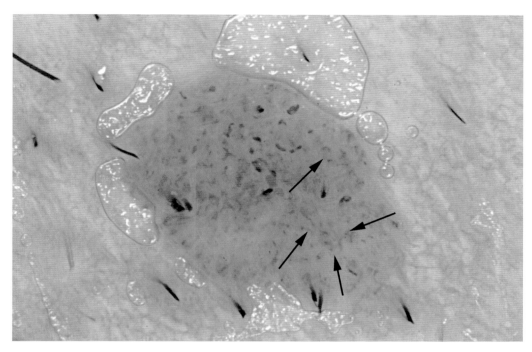

FIGURE 2.90 Telangiectases—comma vessels
Comma vessels (arrows) that appear "C" or comma shaped are found in 66% of dermal or congenital nevi and are highly specific for benign nevi. Only 1% and 2.9% of amelanotic/hypomelanotic melanomas have regularly distributed comma vessels and comma vessels as the predominant vessel type, respectively.

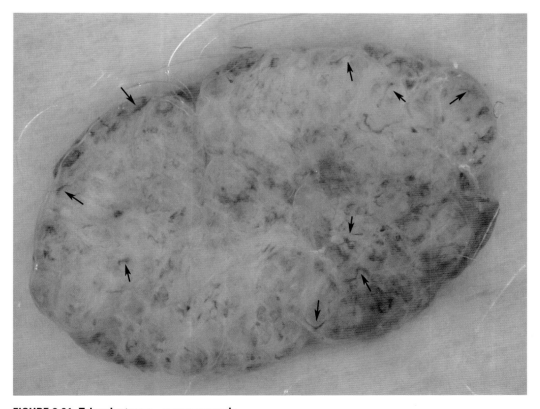

FIGURE 2.91 Telangiectases—comma vessels
Comma vessels are seen as the predominant vessel type in this dermal nevus (arrows).

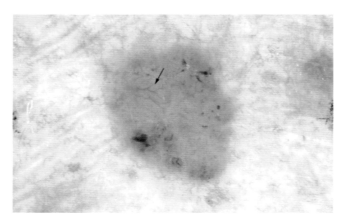

FIGURE 2.92 Telangiectases—arborizing
Arborizing (tree-like) telangiectases are seen with distinct branching (arrow). They occur in 52% of pigmented basal cell carcinoma (as seen here) and less commonly in invasive melanoma (23%) and benign pigmented lesions (8%). Only 9% of amelanotic/hypomelanotic melanomas have arborising vessels as the predominant vessel type.

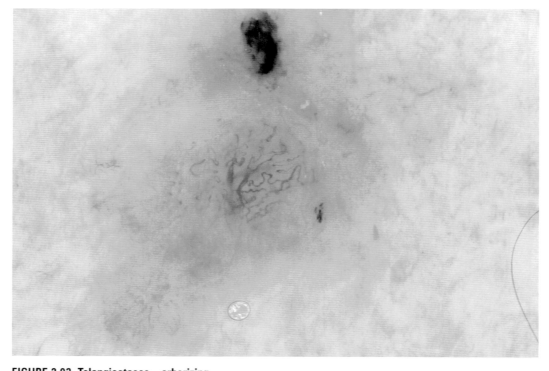

FIGURE 2.93 Telangiectases—arborizing
Here, arborizing vessels are found centrally in this BCC.

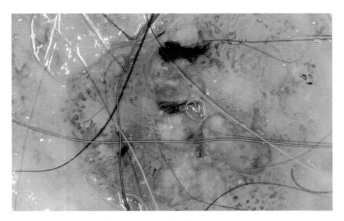

FIGURE 2.94 Telangiectases—hairpin
Hairpin vessels seen as twisting loops are the most frequent vessel found in keratinizing tumors (seborrhoeic keratosis, squamous cell carcinoma, keratoacanthoma). As seen here, telangiectases can occur as regularly distributed loops in seborrheic keratoses.

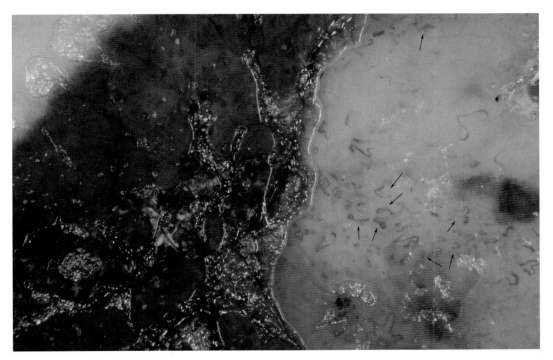

FIGURE 2.95 Telangiectases—hairpin
When found in melanocytic tumors, hairpin vessels (arrows) are a significant feature of melanoma, with 21% of amelanotic/hypomelanotic melanoma having hairpin vessels.

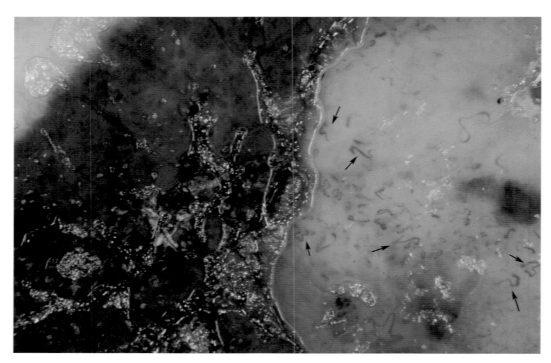

FIGURE 2.96 Telangiectases—linear irregular

Linear irregular vessels (arrows) that are seen as irregular wave-like vessels without branching are a significant feature of melanoma particularly when they are the predominant vessel type (34% sensitivity and 80% specificity for amelanotic/hypomelanotic melanoma).

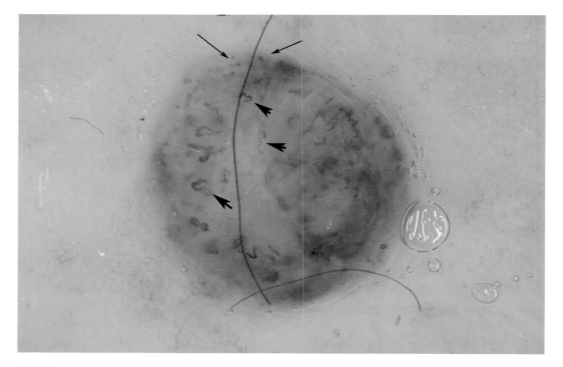

FIGURE 2.97 Telangiectases—linear irregular

Linear irregular vessels (thick arrows) are a more specific feature of melanoma when found in combination with dotted vessels (thin arrows) within a lesion (30% sensitivity and 85% specificity for amelanotic/hypomelanotic melanoma).

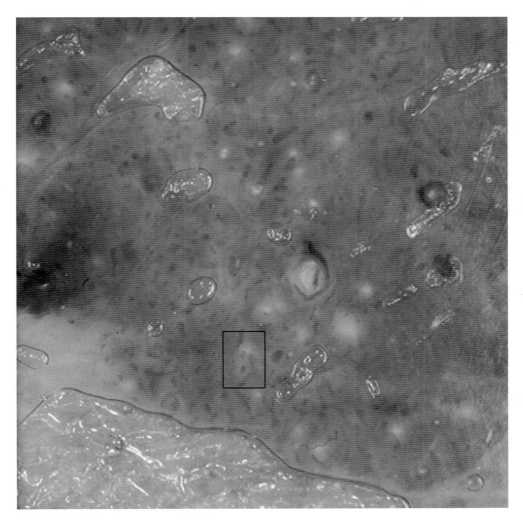

FIGURE 2.98 Telangiectases—white halo

In keratinizing tumors vessels are often surrounded by a white halo (halo vessels; seen within the box).

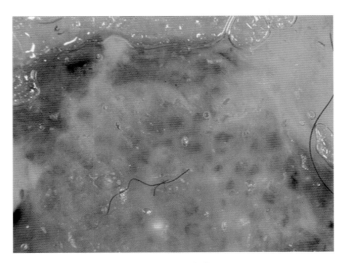

FIGURE 2.99 Telangiectases—white halo

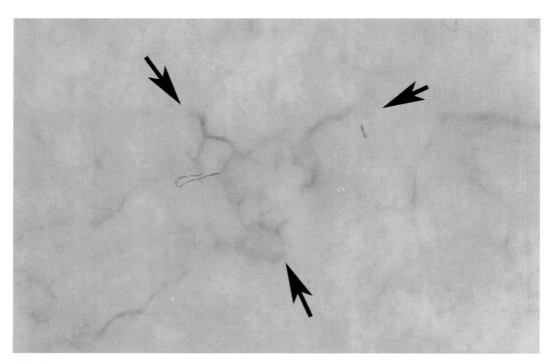

FIGURE 2.100 Telangiectases—crown
Crown vessels, which are seen as orderly, bending, scarcely branching vessels disappearing at the centre of the lesion, are found in sebaceous hyperplasia.

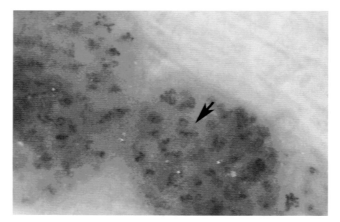

FIGURE 2.101 Telangiectases—winding (cork screw)**
Winding (cork screw) vessels (arrow) are typically found in melanoma metastases.

**This photograph was kindly provided by Dr Riccardo Bono, Rome, Italy.

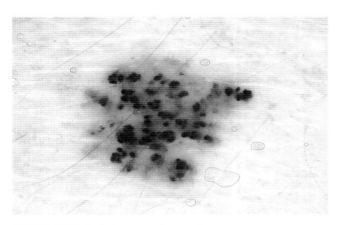

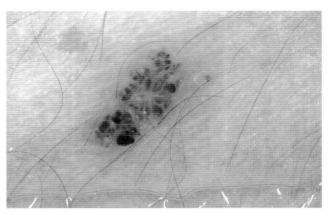

FIGURE 2.102 Red-blue areas (lacunes)

Red-blue areas (lacunes) are sharply demarcated, ovoid structures which may appear as red or red-blue in color (see also Figure 2.40). When many are present in a lesion, they are pathognomonic for hemangiomas. Histopathologically they represent dilated vascular spaces in the dermis.

FIGURE 2.103 Red-blue areas (lacunes)

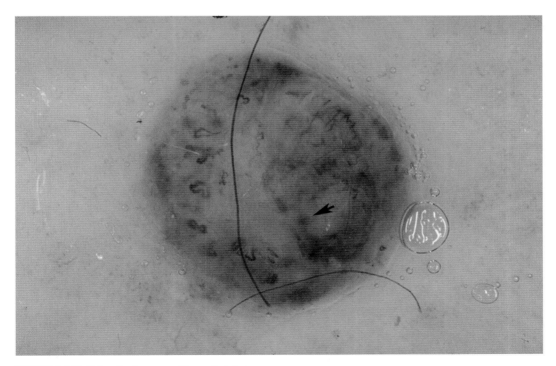

FIGURE 2.104 Telangiectases—milky red globules

Milky red globules (arrow) which are seen as unfocussed (in contrast to red-blue lacunes) red-pink globular structures are overall a significant feature of amelanotic/hypomelanotic melanoma. However, they are not present in a significantly different frequency between melanoma and benign amelanotic/hypomelanotic melanocytic lesions. Diagnosis: Nodular melanoma.

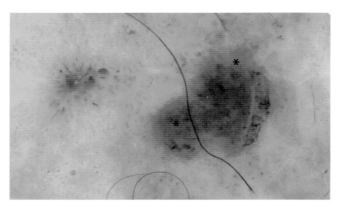

FIGURE 2.105 Milky red areas and greater than one shade of pink
A variant of erythema is milky red areas (asterisks). Here, erythema with an overlying milky film-like area has a sensitivity of 51% and specificity of 71% for amelanotic/hypomelanotic melanoma. A related feature also seen here is more than one shade of pink color which has a 32% sensitivity and 83% specificity for amelanotic/hypomelanotic melanoma. Diagnosis: Invasive melanoma.

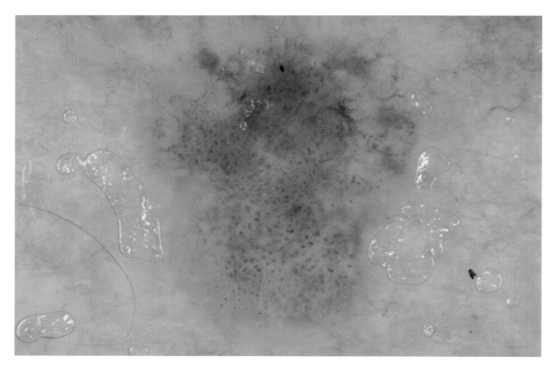

FIGURE 2.106 Predominant central vessels
Here the majority of vessels (in this case dotted) are in a predominantly central position within the lesion. The most significant vascular feature of amelanotic/hypomelanotic melanoma is telangiectasia found predominantly in a central versus peripheral position (predominant central vessels). This feature has a 16% sensitivity and 94% specificity for amelanotic/hypomelanotic melanoma. Diagnosis: Invasive melanoma.

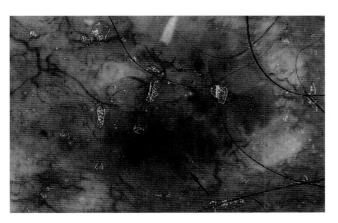

FIGURE 2.107 Leaf-like areas

Leaf-like areas (arrow) are seen as brown to gray/blue discrete bulbous extensions arising almost exclusively in pigmented basal cell carcinomas (as seen here). They should be distinguished from pseudopods because the bulbous projections of maple leaf-like areas are discrete pigmented nests, never arising from a network and usually not arising from a confluent pigmented tumor.

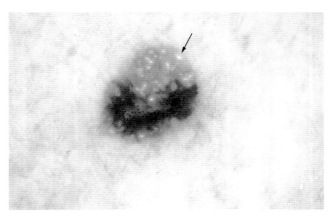

FIGURE 2.109 Milia-like cysts

Milia-like cysts are seen as discrete, white or yellow, opalescent, round bodies within the body of a lesion. They are commonly seen in seborrheic keratoses, with multiple large milia-like cysts being almost pathognomonic for this lesion. They also are seen not uncommonly in compound or dermal nevi (particularly congenital nevi). Solitary or a few milia-like cysts can occur in melanoma, pigmented BCC, and less commonly in other pigmented lesions. Only 1% of amelanotic/hypomelanotic melanoma have four or more milia-like cysts. The arrow indicates multiple white milia cysts in a seborrheic keratosis.

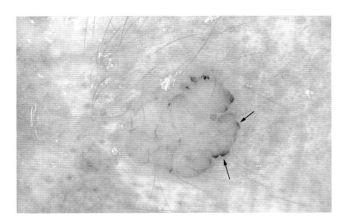

FIGURE 2.108 Leaf-like areas

The arrows indicate leaf areas in a pigmented basal cell carcinoma.

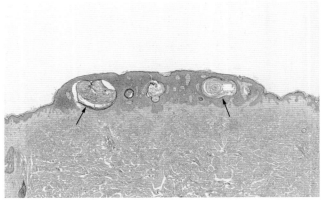

FIGURE 2.110 Milia-like cysts—histopathology

Histopathologically milia-like cysts represent intraepidermal keratin cysts (arrows). This is a section from the seborrheic keratosis in Figure 2.109. Magnification ×8 (H & E stain).

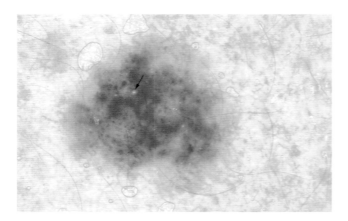

FIGURE 2.111 Milia-like cysts in a congenital compound nevus
See also Figure 2.119 for an example of milia cysts in a congenital nevus. Unlike many seborrheic keratoses, when milia cysts are present in other pigmented lesions they are usually only few in number.

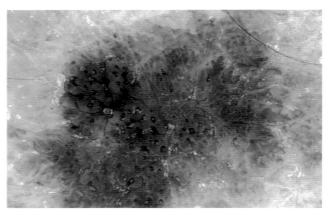

FIGURE 2.113 Fissures and ridges
Fissures are seen as confluent branching clefts in the body of a lesion. In most cases they can be distinguished from the papillomatous clefts of a lesion by their greater width (see Figure 2.27). The raised structures between fissures are called ridges. Fissures and ridges are seen primarily in seborrheic keratoses, but occur also in compound and dermal nevi (usually the congenital variety). Less commonly, fissures are found in melanoma and other pigmented lesions. This lesion is a seborrheic keratosis.

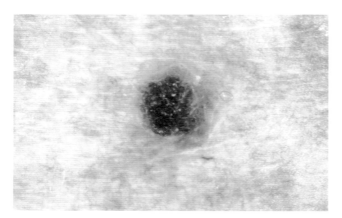

FIGURE 2.112 Keratin
The reason for using liquid on the skin in dermoscopy is that it removes the reflection of light from the stratum corneum. Hence surface scale essentially disappears. However, when focally increased, scale (keratin) can be seen as a white/pale yellow crystalline (reflective) surface. It occurs commonly in pigmented solar keratoses and seborrheic keratoses, and is not infrequently found in melanoma (and less commonly in other melanocytic lesions). This lesion is a pigmented solar keratosis, with keratin seen as a white crystalline structure throughout the lesion.

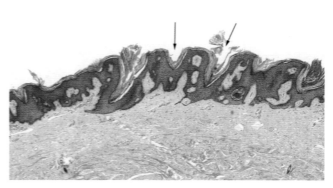

FIGURE 2.114 Fissures—histopathology
This section from the lesion in Figure 2.113 shows the fissures as wedge-shaped clefts (arrows). Magnification ×10 (H & E stain).

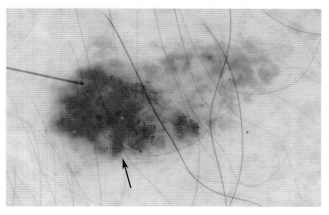

FIGURE 2.115 Fat fingers

When ridges are enlarged or separated by larger width fissures they can form linear, curvilinear, round/oval or branched "fat fingers" (arrow) as seen in some pigmented seborrheic keratoses.

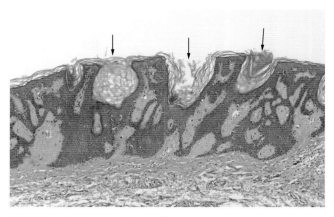

FIGURE 2.117 Crypts—histopathology

Histopathologically crypts are concave, often hyperkeratinized clefts. They are a morphological variant of fissures. This section is of the lesion in Figure 2.116. Magnification ×25 (H & E stain).

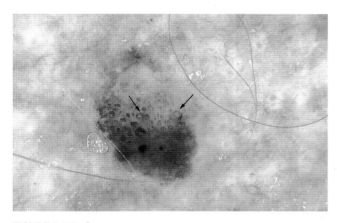

FIGURE 2.116 Crypts

Crypts (comedo-like openings) appear as irregularly shaped craters (arrows). Like fissures they are seen primarily in seborrheic keratoses, but occur also in compound and dermal nevi (usually the congenital variety). They are rarely seen in melanoma. This lesion is a seborrheic keratosis.

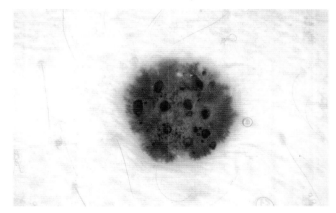

FIGURE 2.118 Crypts in a seborrheic keratosis

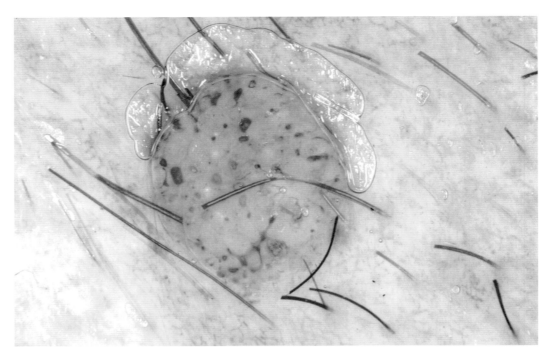

FIGURE 2.119 Crypts and fissures in a congenital dermal nevus
This congenital dermal nevus contains predominantly crypts with some fissures. It is morphologically indistinguishable from a seborrheic keratosis. Note the milia cysts also present. Clinically it may be distinguished from a seborrheic keratosis by its soft consistency.

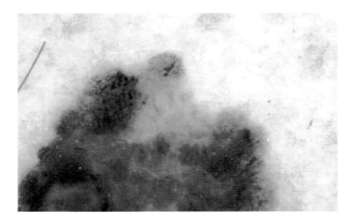

FIGURE 2.120 Irregular depigmentation
The finding of depigmentation may indicate histopathological regression in pigmented lesions. Depigmentation found at any site within a lesion is a significant feature of invasive melanoma, but it lacks adequate specificity to be a clinically useful discriminant. However, an irregular pattern of depigmentation (irregular depigmentation) is more specific, with a specificity of 92% and a sensitivity of 46% for invasive melanoma. This lesion is an invasive melanoma.

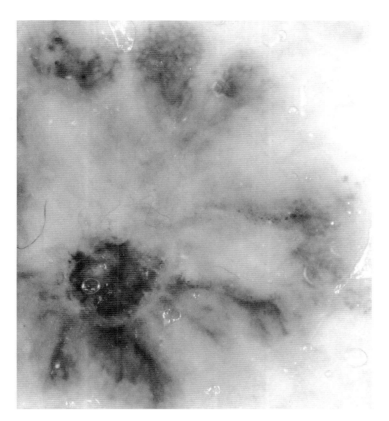

FIGURE 2.121 Irregular depigmentation in an invasive melanoma
Histopathological regression is a common feature of superficial spreading melanoma.
It presents as irregular depigmentation extending to the periphery in this melanoma.
Note that while large areas of regression have occurred in this lesion, the presence
of an obvious network confirms its melanocytic origin.

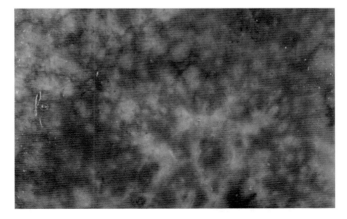

FIGURE 2.122 Scar-like depigmentation
The presence of scar-like depigmentation is a significant feature of invasive
melanoma, with a specificity of 93% and a sensitivity of 36%. It is seen
as white or near white reticular extensions, as in this lentigo maligna
melanoma.

FIGURE 2.123 Scar-like depigmentation in an invasive melanoma
Gross regression in this melanoma is seen with areas of irregular and scar-like depigmentation.

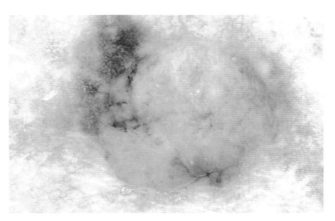

FIGURE 2.124 Depigmented (amelanotic/hypomelanotic) nodule
Depigmentation can be found in non-regressing lesions as a consequence of an absence of pigmented cells (e.g. as seen in the dermal component of many melanocytic nevi, or the amelanotic nodules of melanoma). Here, a depigmented nodule constituting the dermal component of a compound nevus is seen.

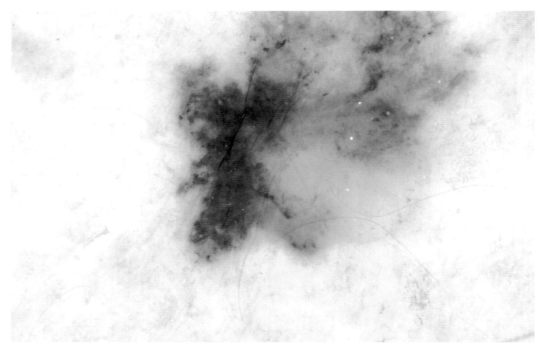

FIGURE 2.125 Depigmented (amelanotic) nodule in a melanoma
The amelanotic nodules of melanoma tend to be more vascular than in benign lesions. Here, dotted and small hairpin telangiectases are seen exclusively in the hypomelanotic nodule of a superficial spreading melanoma (see also Figure 2.95).

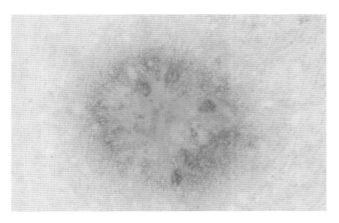

FIGURE 2.126 White scar-like patch
This is seen as a white stellate (star shaped) area normally found in a central position (as seen here) in more than half of dermatofibromas.

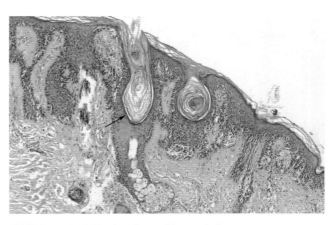

FIGURE 2.128 Follicular plugs—histopathology
The arrow indicates a follicular plug (keratin-filled hair follicle). Magnification ×25 (H & E stain).

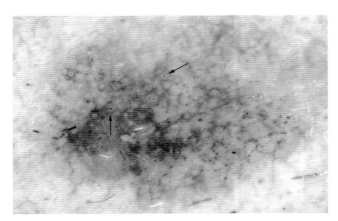

FIGURE 2.127 Follicular plugs
Follicular plugs are seen as well-defined round "target" structures. They can be found on normal skin, particularly on the face, where they can form a "pseudo-network" pattern, with the follicular plugs constituting the holes of the network and the remaining interfollicular pigment forming the grids (cords). The arrows indicate follicular plugs in a dysplastic nevus on the face.

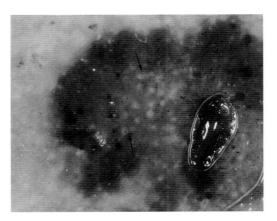

FIGURE 2.129 Follicular plugs in a melanoma
Follicular plugs are a significant feature of invasive melanoma. This lesion is an invasive melanoma on the face.

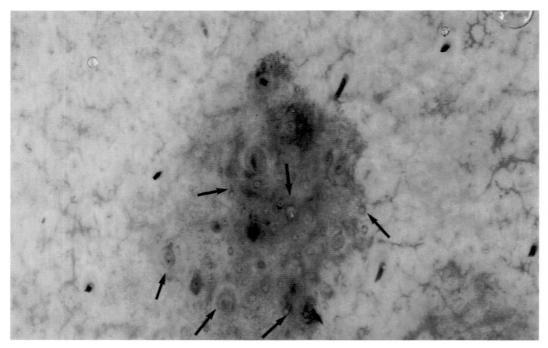

FIGURE 2.130
Asymmetric pigmented follicular openings

Asymmetric pigmented follicular openings refer to dark pigmentation in an asymmetric distribution around follicular openings (arrows). They are formed by an asymmetric descent of melanoma cells within individual hair follicles. They are seen in 68% of lentigo maligna but only 12% of benign pigmented macules of the face.

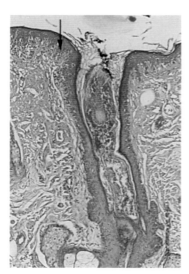

FIGURE 2.131 Asymmetric pigmented follicular openings—histopathology

In lentigo maligna there are atypical melanocytes concentrated in the basal layer of the epidermis which extend down the follicular epithelium of the hairs. In this case there are more melanocytes on one side (arrow) of the upper follicular epithelium compared with the other side. This variation in melanocyte concentration leads to asymmetry in the pigment pattern of follicular openings. Magnification ×10 (H & E stain).

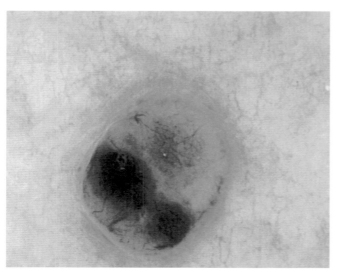

FIGURE 2.132 Large blue-gray ovoid nests

Large blue-gray ovoid nests are well-circumscribed, confluent or near confluent pigmented ovoid or elongated areas, larger than globules, and not intimately connected to a pigmented tumor body. They are the single most useful feature for the diagnosis of pigmented basal cell carcinoma, with 55% of pigmented BCC having this feature but only 3% of melanoma and 1% of benign pigmented lesions.

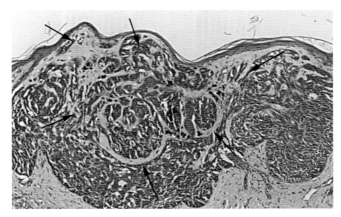

FIGURE 2.133 Large blue-gray ovoid nests—histopathology
In this basal cell carcinoma the melanin pigment is concentrated within a large nest of tumor cells (delineated by arrows). Magnification ×50 (H & E stain).

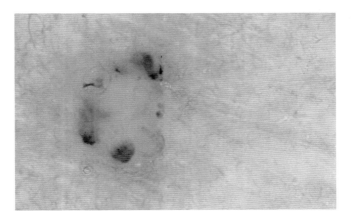

FIGURE 2.134 Large blue-gray ovoid nests in a pigmented BCC

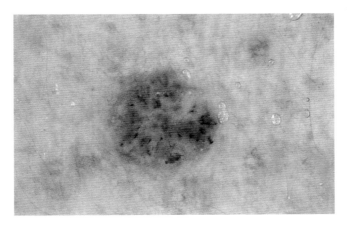

FIGURE 2.135 Multiple blue-gray globules
Multiple blue-gray globules should be differentiated from multiple blue-gray dots by their larger size and well-circumscribed morphology. They are a highly specific feature (97%) for pigmented basal cell carcinoma and occur in 27% of these lesions.

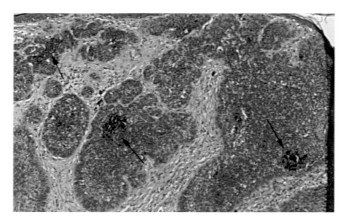

FIGURE 2.136 Multiple blue-gray globules——histopathology
There are scattered focal collections of melanin pigment within the tumor nests of basal cell carcinoma (arrows). These collections are smaller than seen in Figure 2.133. Magnification ×50 (H & E stain).

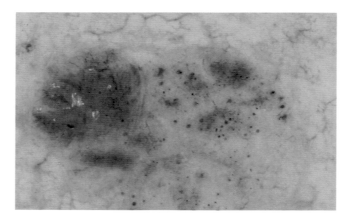

FIGURE 2.137 Multiple blue-gray globules in a pigmented BCC
While some of these globules are small, they lack the "pepper-like" morphology seen with multiple blue-gray dots (see Figures 2.59, 2.61).

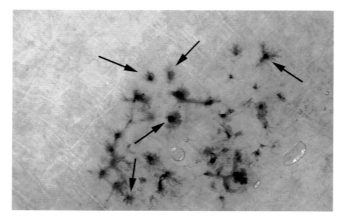

FIGURE 2.138 Spoke wheel areas
Spoke wheel areas are well-circumscribed radial projections, usually tan but sometimes blue or gray, meeting at an often darker central axis (arrows). They are highly specific (100%) for pigmented basal cell carcinoma, but found in only 10% of these lesions.

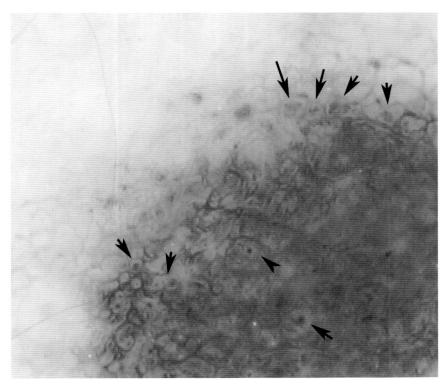

FIGURE 2.139 Target globules (magnified view)
Target globules are seen as brown to blue globules with a surrounding white halo. They are found more frequently in congenital nevi.

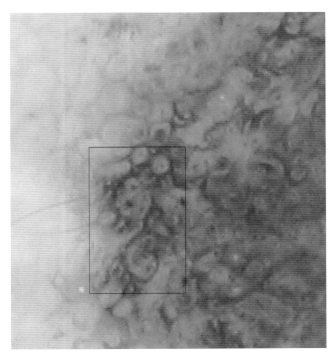

FIGURE 2.140 Target network (magnified view)
Here a normal pigmented network surrounds target globules. This feature is also found more frequently in congenital nevi.

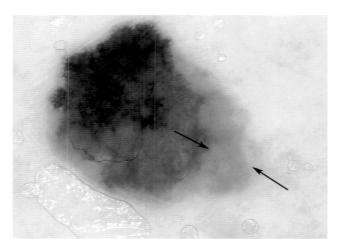

FIGURE 2.141 Peripheral light-brown structureless areas

Peripheral light-brown structureless areas (delineated by the arrows) is seen as light-brown variable sized and shaped areas found at the periphery of a lesion and occupying more than 10% of its surface. This feature has a sensitivity of 63% and specificity of 96% for the diagnosis of thin melanoma, and a 19% sensitivity and 93% specificity for the diagnosis of hypomelanotic melanoma.

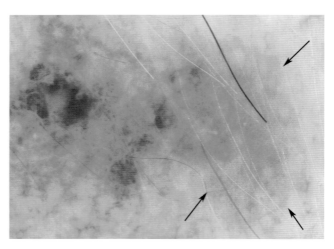

FIGURE 2.143 Peripheral light-brown structureless areas

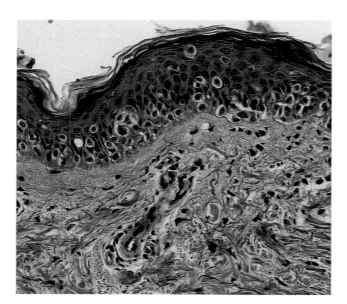

FIGURE 2.142 Peripheral light-brown structureless areas—histopathology

Histologically, peripheral light-brown structureless areas are due to relative flattening of the rete ridges in combination with a preponderance of single cell pagetoid melanoma cells and pigmented keratinocytes rather than the formation of nests in the epidermis.

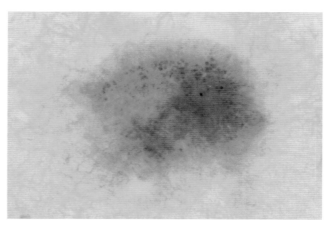

FIGURE 2.144 Peripheral light-brown structureless areas

CHAPTER THREE

BENIGN PIGMENTED MACULES

Ephelis (freckle)

An ephelis is a solar-induced pigmented macule (flat lesion) that has a normal number of melanocytes producing an increased amount of melanin. Under dermoscopy the ephelis has the following features:

- uniform pigmented background (majority)
- moth-eaten edge (common)
- absent brown globules

Solar lentigo

The solar lentigo is histologically defined as having actinic dermal changes, elongated rete ridges and usually a normal number of melanocytes producing an increased amount of melanin. The dermoscopic features are:

- discrete (lightly pigmented) regular network (common)
- fingerprint-like structures (some)
- uniform pigmented background (some)
- absent brown globules

Under dermoscopy, the elongated rete ridges often lead to the appearance of a pigmented network, thus distinguishing the solar lentigo from the ephelis. However, the ephelis and the solar lentigo can overlap in their dermoscopic morphology.

Lentigo simplex (ink spot lentigo)

The lentigo simplex has an increased number of melanocytes producing increased melanin. The lentigo simplex characteristically has a uniform distinct network occupying the entire lesion. The surface microscopic features are:

- uniform pigmented network (majority)
- prominent (darkly pigmented) regular network (common)
- areas of blue pigmentation (some)
- absent brown globules

Dermal melanophages can be seen in any of the above melanocytic-derived lesions, particularly in the lentigo simplex. Depending on their density, they are seen as blue dots/globules or confluent blue areas under dermoscopy.

Pigmented solar keratosis

Pigmented solar keratoses are morphologically variable under dermoscopy. They have varying degrees of keratin/scale, which is often not apparent under the surface microscope because of the application of liquid. Furthermore, when on the face they commonly have a pseudo-broadened discrete network due to the presence of hair follicles, which form the hypodense "holes" of the network. Their dermoscopic features are:

- keratin/scale (common)
- tan uniform pigmented background (common)
- discrete/regular pseudo-broadened network (when on the face) (some)
- broken areas of pseudo-broadened network (when on the face) (some)
- absent fissures/ridges, crypts, milia-like cysts (majority)

In some cases pigmented actinic keratoses of the face can mimic lentigo maligna, with rhomboidal structures and multiple blue-gray dots forming annular granular patterns.[1] In contrast, non-pigmented facial actinic keratoses show a "strawberry" appearance of red pseudo-network composed of erythema and linear-wavy telangiectasia between follicular openings (sometimes with yellow follicular plugs) surrounded by a white halo.[2]

References

1. Zalaudek, I, Ferrara, G, Leinweber, B, Mercogliano, A, D'Ambrosio, A, Argenziano, G. Pitfalls in the clinical and dermoscopic diagnosis of pigmented actinic keratosis. *J Am Acad Dermatol* 2005; 53:1071–4.

2. Zalaudek, I, Giacomel, J, Argenziano, G, Hofmann-Wellenhof, R, Micantonio, T, Di Stefani, A, Oliviero, M, Rabinovitz, H, Soyer, HP, Peris, K. Dermoscopy of facial nonpigmented actinic keratosis. *Br J Dermatol* 2006; 155: 951–6.

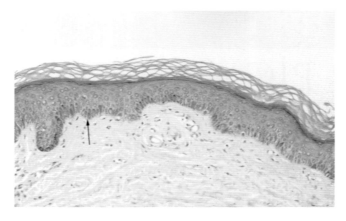

FIGURE 3.1 Ephelis/freckle (histopathology)
This ephelis shows the characteristic basal pigmentation (arrow). The pigment is in keratinocytes. There is no increase in melanocytes and the architecture of the epidermis is normal. Magnification ×50 (H & E stain).

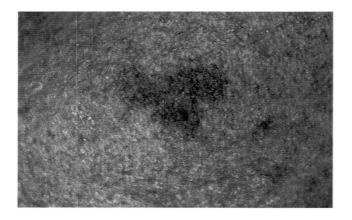

FIGURE 3.2 (a) Ephelis/freckle (clinical view)
The ephelis is seen as a solar-induced pigmented macule (flat lesion).

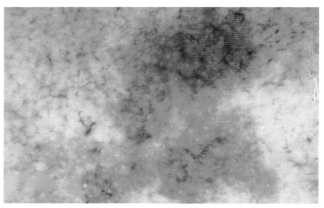

FIGURE 3.2 (b) Ephelis/freckle (dermoscopy)
A characteristic finding of the ephelis under dermoscopy is a uniform tan background of pigmentation and a lack of discrete brown globules.

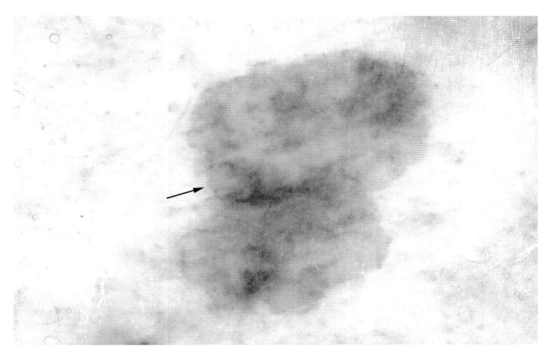

FIGURE 3.3 Ephelis/freckle (dermoscopy)
This lesion has the classic dermoscopic features of a uniform pigmented background, areas of moth-eaten edge (arrow) and a lack of brown globules.

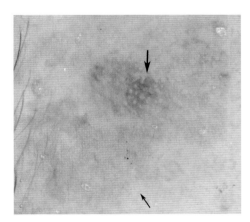

FIGURE 3.4 Ephelis/freckle (dermoscopy)
This lesion has a large area of uniform pigment background with an area of moth-eaten edge (thin arrow). In addition there is a focal area of pseudo-broadened network due to the follicular openings of the face (thick arrow).

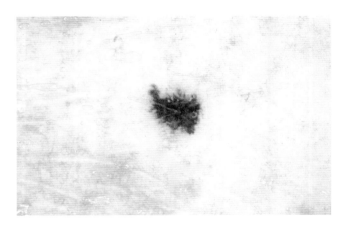

FIGURE 3.5 Ephelis/freckle (dermoscopy)
While the majority of freckles are tan in color, some have uniform, prominent pigmentation.

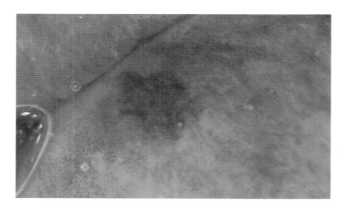

FIGURE 3.6 Ephelis/freckle—lip (dermoscopy)

This lesion on the lower vermilion lip has symmetrical pigmentation pattern. There is an overlap in the morphology of these lesions with melanotic macules on the vermilion lip.

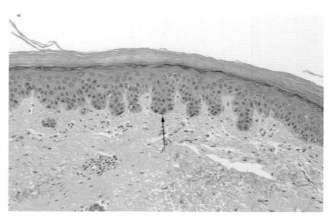

FIGURE 3.7 Solar lentigo (histopathology)

The solar lentigo characteristically has elongation of the epidermal rete ridges (arrow), an increase in basal pigmentation, but no increase in melanocytes. The underlying dermis shows solar elastosis. Magnification ×50 (H & E stain).

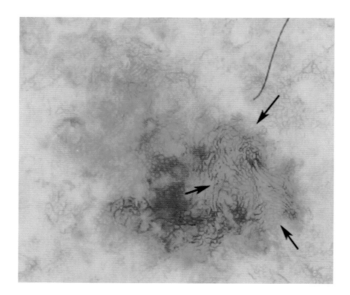

FIGURE 3.8 Solar lentigo (dermoscopy)

Under dermoscopy the elongated rete ridges often lead to the appearance of a pigment network (as seen here), thus distinguishing the solar lentigo from the ephelis. Fingerprint-like structures are seen as curvilinear structures (the area delineated by the arrows). However, the ephelis and solar lentigo can overlap in their dermoscopic morphology. Like the ephelis, the solar lentigo lacks conspicuous brown globules, thus differentiating it from many junctional nevi.

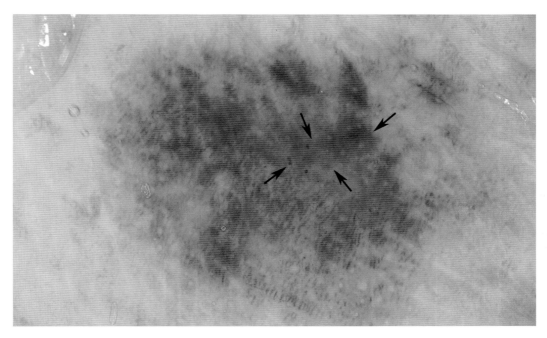

FIGURE 3.9 Solar lentigo (dermoscopy)
This lesion shows areas of linear fingerprint-like areas (inferior half of the lesion) and a focus of early seborrheic keratosis with small crypts and milia (delineated by the arrows). Many solar lentigo transform into seborrheic keratoses.

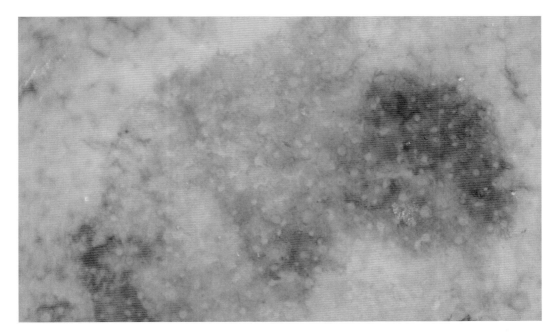

FIGURE 3.10 Solar lentigo (dermoscopy)
This lesion shows a uniform pigment background in between the round follicular openings. In contrast to lentigo maligna, the majority of these follicular openings show uniform pigmentation around their rim without asymmetric clumping. This lesion can only be distinguished from an ephelis by histopathological examination.

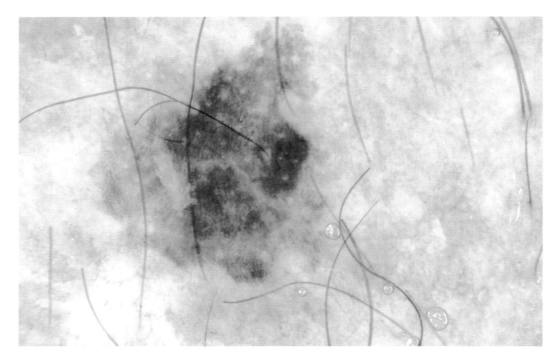

FIGURE 3.11 Solar lentigo (dermoscopy)

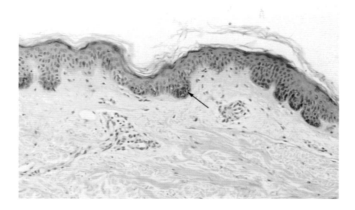

FIGURE 3.12 Lentigo simplex (histopathology)
The lentigo simplex has elongated rete ridges, increased basal pigmentation with an increase in melanocytes (arrow). Unlike melanocytic nevi, no nesting of melanocytes is seen. Melanocytes have a smaller nucleus than the surrounding keratinocytes and have pale cytoplasm which often shrinks, leaving a clearing around the cell. Magnification ×50 (H & E stain).

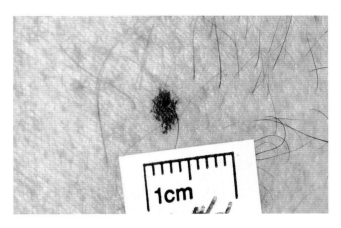

FIGURE 3.13 (a) Lentigo simplex (clinical view)
In this common presentation of lentigo simplex, a dark brown to black discrete macule is seen.

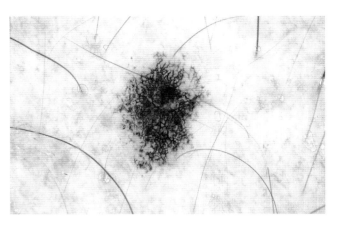

FIGURE 3.13 (b) Lentigo simplex (dermoscopy)
Classically, the lentigo simplex is seen as having a prominent (darkly pigmented) network occupying its entire surface.

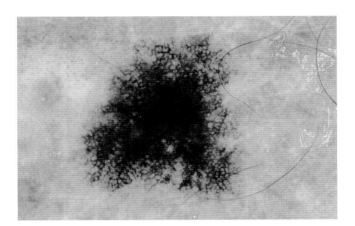

FIGURE 3.14 Lentigo simplex (dermoscopy)
Unlike junctional nevi, the lentigo simplex lacks brown globules (nests of melanocytes at or near the dermoepidermal junction).

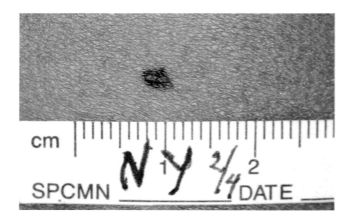

FIGURE 3.15 (a) Lentigo simplex (clinical view)
The lentigo simplex can be one of the most heavily pigmented lesions seen.

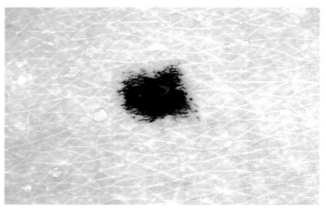

FIGURE 3.15 (b) Lentigo simplex (dermoscopy)
However, the uniform, prominent (ink-black) network confirms the diagnosis. Note that when pigmentation is excessively dense, areas of the network are less clearly defined.

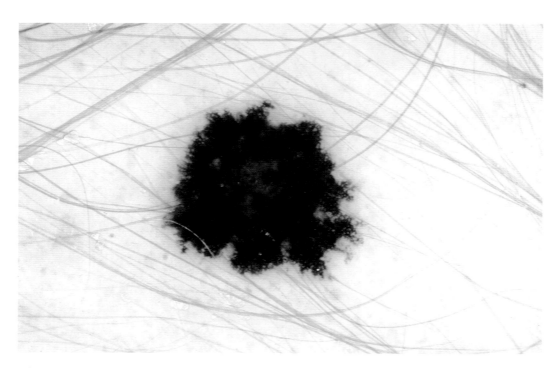

FIGURE 3.16 Lentigo simplex (dermoscopy)
Areas of confluent blue pigment, mimicking blue-white veil, are seen in this lesion. This lead to excision of the lesion. However, the only other dermoscopic feature seen is a uniform ink-black network. This confirms the diagnosis of lentigo simplex. The blue pigmentation is due to dense accumulation of melanophages (melanin-laden macrophages) which are commonly found in lentigo simplex.

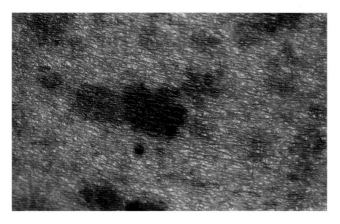

FIGURE 3.17 (a) Lentigo simplex (clinical view)
Not all of these lentigines are darkly pigmented. Note the presence of distinct skin markings, which should never be lost in lentigo simplex.

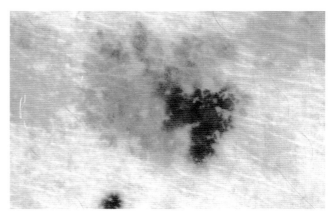

FIGURE 3.17 (b) Lentigo simplex (dermoscopy)
In this variant of lentigo simplex only uniform background pigmentation is seen.

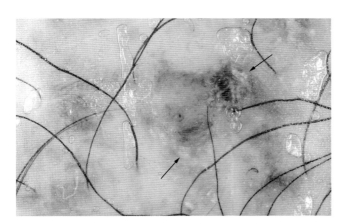

FIGURE 3.18 Pigmented solar keratosis (dermoscopy)
Pigmented solar keratoses are morphologically variable under dermoscopy. A common presentation is a lesion with a uniform tan-pigmented background with focal keratin/scale (arrows). The majority lack distinct fissures/ridges, crypts and milia-like cysts, thus differentiating them from seborrheic keratoses.

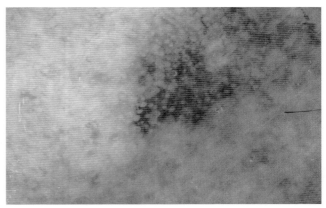

FIGURE 3.19 Pigmented solar keratosis (dermoscopy)
Pigmented solar keratoses have varying degrees of keratin/scale, which is often not apparent under the surface microscope because of the application of liquid. Furthermore, when on the face they commonly have a pseudo-broadened network due to the presence of hair follicles which form the hypodense "holes" of the network. This lesion can only be distinguished from a lentigo by histopathology.

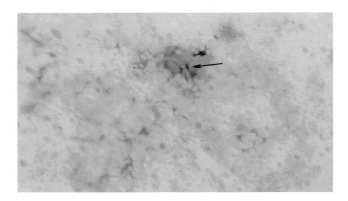

FIGURE 3.20 Pigmented solar keratosis (dermoscopy)
This lesion has areas of broken pseudo-broadened network (arrow) characteristic of some pigmented facial solar keratoses.

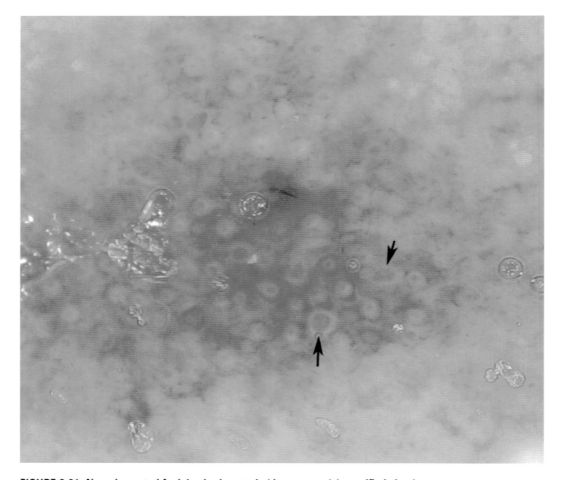

FIGURE 3.21 Non-pigmented facial solar keratosis (dermoscopy) (magnified view)
In contrast, non-pigmented facial solar keratoses show a "strawberry" appearance of red pseudo-network composed of erythema and linear-wavy telangiectasia between follicular openings (sometimes with yellow follicular plugs such as indicated by the arrows) surrounded by a white halo.

CHAPTER FOUR

MELANOCYTIC NEVI

Common benign acquired nevi (moles)

These lesions are formed from proliferating cells derived from melanocytes (nevus cells). They are categorized by the position of these cells in the skin. In general, the dermoscopy global patterns of these banal acquired nevi show a symmetrical pattern involving any of the three basic elements: network, globules, and homogeneous pigmentation.[1–2] The proportion of these elements differ with nevus type (junctional, compound, or dermal as detailed below) and age.

Globular patterns are more frequent in childhood and network (reticular) patterns more frequent in adults.[3] In skin type 1 individuals (who never tan following sun exposure), nevi are predominantly light brown in color, often with central hypopigmentation, whereas dark brown nevi become increasingly common as skin type increases (easier ability to tan). In skin type IV individuals (rarely burns) nevi with central increased pigmentation are common.[4] Finally, within individuals, repeated global patterns of nevi are often seen.[5,6]

Junctional nevi

Junctional nevi are composed of nests of nevus cells at the dermoepidermal junction. They are discrete, flat, pigmented lesions that have the dermoscopic features of:

- relatively regular/discrete network (majority)
- graduated regular edge (common)
- symmetrical pigmentation pattern (common)
- black dots/globules (uncommon or rarely seen)

Compound nevi

Compound nevi have nevus cells both at the dermoepidermal junction and in the dermis. They have the dermoscopic features of:

- areas of regular/discrete network (common)
- areas of uniform homogeneous pigmentation (common)
- graduated edge (common)

- symmetrical pigmentation pattern (common)
- regular depigmentation, often central (common)
- brown globules, uniform in shape and size (common)

Whether a compound nevus has a majority of its lesion containing a network, rather than areas of homogeneous pigmentation, depends on the relative amounts of junctional and dermal components (i.e. the network is formed by the junctional component and the homogeneous pigmentation by the dermal component). Indeed, it is not uncommon for compound nevi to lack the presence of a network when the junctional component is sparse.

Dermal nevi

The dermal nevus is formed entirely by nevus cells in the dermis. Following a general principle of dermoscopy that *associates increasing depth of pathology in the skin with a decrease in morphological definition,* dermal nevi are relatively structureless. The features of dermal nevi are:

- absent network, brown and black dots/globules (universal)
- faint homogeneous pigmentation (common)
- comma vessels (common)
- amelanotic (some)
- papillomatous cobblestone pattern (some)

While dermal nevi can contain telangiectases, they are generally less vascular than amelanotic nodules of invasive melanoma and nodular BCCs. Comma vessels, preferentially found at the periphery, are the most frequently found telangiectasia in dermal nevi.

Congenital nevi

Congenital melanocytic nevi are present at birth and are classified by their size: small (<1.5 cm diameter), intermediate (1.5–20 cm) or large (>20 cm). Under dermoscopy examination they tend to have more structures than benign non-congenital acquired nevi.[7] Furthermore, they have the

following features more frequently seen than non-congenital benign nevi: globular pattern, increased number of hair follicles, loss of pigment in the skin furrows, focal broadening of the network, target network, target globules, and vascular structures.[7] The dermoscopic features of congenital nevi are:[7-9]

- pigment network (common)
- globules (common)
- homogeneous pigmentation (common)
- hair follicles (often with surrounding depigmentation) (common)
- milia-like cysts (common)
- skin furrow hypopigmentation (common)
- vessels (common)
- target globules (some)
- target network (some)
- focal broadened network (some)

Like all nevi, loss of pigment around the hair follicles (perifollicular depigmentation) can be seen. Finally, both age and site can influence the dermoscopic appearance of congenital nevi, with globular patterns more frequent in childhood and reticular patterns preferentially seen on the limbs.[7,8]

Halo nevi

Halo nevi present as peripherally regressing benign nevi most commonly seen in adolescence and preferentially on the trunk.[10] Under dermoscopy examination the central nevus most frequently has either a globular or homogeneous pigmentation pattern without specific features for melanoma. When followed over time, an increase in the white halo with diminution of the central nevus is commonly seen. Since a circumferential white halo is very rarely seen in melanoma (0.4%), and when present other specific dermoscopic features for melanoma may be visualized, a confident diagnosis of halo nevi as benign is usually easily made.[10]

Recurrent nevi

Pigmentation in a scar following removal of a melanocytic lesion can be due to a true recurrence of the lesion or reactive pigment changes without proliferation of melanocytes.[11] While there can be a morphological overlap between these under dermoscopic examination, the presence of globules or a heterogeneous pattern favor a true recurrence of the lesion.[11] The management of recurrent nevi, while depending upon the original pathology, can be assisted by short-term digital dermoscopy monitoring, with lack of change after 3 months leading to observation (see Chapter 8).

Acral lentiginous nevi

Nevi on volar sites (palms or soles) have a distinct morphology that differs from nevi on non-volar body sites. While a number of variations have been described, the basic element of acral nevi is the parallel furrow pattern with its histopathological correlation of nevus cells found in the crista profunda limitans, an epidermal rete ridge underlying the surface furrow (see Chapter 2).[12] Depending upon the anatomical site on the sole of the foot the parallel furrow pattern may remain intact (non-arch), show a lattice-like pattern (arch) or fibrillar-filamentous pattern (weight bearing surface).[13] The dermoscopic features of acral nevi are[12-16]:

- symmetry of pattern (majority)
- parallel furrow pattern (common)
- lattice-like pattern (some)
- fibrillar-fillamentous pattern (some)
- homogeneous pattern (some)
- globular pattern (some)
- reticular (network) pattern (some)
- globulostreak-like pattern (some)

Depending upon the series, 5–15% of acral nevi show non-typical patterns not described above.[12]

Dysplastic (Clark's) nevi

Dysplastic nevi are melanocytic nevi with cytologic atypia of junctional melanocyte/nevus cells in association with architectural atypia. Melanoma arises from dysplastic nevi more frequently than from common nevi. However, while they can be considered as an intermediate in the spectrum of common benign nevi and melanoma, they are benign. Because of their atypia, they possess greater morphological variability than any other benign pigmented lesion.[1,2,17] The major features of dysplastic nevi are:

- asymmetric pigmentation pattern (common)
- irregularly distributed and shaped brown globules (common)
- network irregular/discrete (common)
- network irregular/prominent (some)
- network edge abrupt (some)
- irregular/graduated edge (common)
- central black dots (some)
- irregular depigmentation (some)

CHAPTER FOUR

MELANOCYTIC NEVI

Common benign acquired nevi (moles)

These lesions are formed from proliferating cells derived from melanocytes (nevus cells). They are categorized by the position of these cells in the skin. In general, the dermoscopy global patterns of these banal acquired nevi show a symmetrical pattern involving any of the three basic elements: network, globules, and homogeneous pigmentation.[1–2] The proportion of these elements differ with nevus type (junctional, compound, or dermal as detailed below) and age.

Globular patterns are more frequent in childhood and network (reticular) patterns more frequent in adults.[3] In skin type 1 individuals (who never tan following sun exposure), nevi are predominantly light brown in color, often with central hypopigmentation, whereas dark brown nevi become increasingly common as skin type increases (easier ability to tan). In skin type IV individuals (rarely burns) nevi with central increased pigmentation are common.[4] Finally, within individuals, repeated global patterns of nevi are often seen.[5,6]

Junctional nevi

Junctional nevi are composed of nests of nevus cells at the dermoepidermal junction. They are discrete, flat, pigmented lesions that have the dermoscopic features of:

- relatively regular/discrete network (majority)
- graduated regular edge (common)
- symmetrical pigmentation pattern (common)
- black dots/globules (uncommon or rarely seen)

Compound nevi

Compound nevi have nevus cells both at the dermoepidermal junction and in the dermis. They have the dermoscopic features of:

- areas of regular/discrete network (common)
- areas of uniform homogeneous pigmentation (common)
- graduated edge (common)
- symmetrical pigmentation pattern (common)
- regular depigmentation, often central (common)
- brown globules, uniform in shape and size (common)

Whether a compound nevus has a majority of its lesion containing a network, rather than areas of homogeneous pigmentation, depends on the relative amounts of junctional and dermal components (i.e. the network is formed by the junctional component and the homogeneous pigmentation by the dermal component). Indeed, it is not uncommon for compound nevi to lack the presence of a network when the junctional component is sparse.

Dermal nevi

The dermal nevus is formed entirely by nevus cells in the dermis. Following a general principle of dermoscopy that *associates increasing depth of pathology in the skin with a decrease in morphological definition,* dermal nevi are relatively structureless. The features of dermal nevi are:

- absent network, brown and black dots/globules (universal)
- faint homogeneous pigmentation (common)
- comma vessels (common)
- amelanotic (some)
- papillomatous cobblestone pattern (some)

While dermal nevi can contain telangiectases, they are generally less vascular than amelanotic nodules of invasive melanoma and nodular BCCs. Comma vessels, preferentially found at the periphery, are the most frequently found telangiectasia in dermal nevi.

Congenital nevi

Congenital melanocytic nevi are present at birth and are classified by their size: small (<1.5 cm diameter), intermediate (1.5–20 cm) or large (>20 cm). Under dermoscopy examination they tend to have more structures than benign non-congenital acquired nevi.[7] Furthermore, they have the

following features more frequently seen than non-congenital benign nevi: globular pattern, increased number of hair follicles, loss of pigment in the skin furrows, focal broadening of the network, target network, target globules, and vascular structures.[7] The dermoscopic features of congenital nevi are:[7–9]

- pigment network (common)
- globules (common)
- homogeneous pigmentation (common)
- hair follicles (often with surrounding depigmentation) (common)
- milia-like cysts (common)
- skin furrow hypopigmentation (common)
- vessels (common)
- target globules (some)
- target network (some)
- focal broadened network (some)

Like all nevi, loss of pigment around the hair follicles (perifollicular depigmentation) can be seen. Finally, both age and site can influence the dermoscopic appearance of congenital nevi, with globular patterns more frequent in childhood and reticular patterns preferentially seen on the limbs.[7,8]

Halo nevi

Halo nevi present as peripherally regressing benign nevi most commonly seen in adolescence and preferentially on the trunk.[10] Under dermoscopy examination the central nevus most frequently has either a globular or homogeneous pigmentation pattern without specific features for melanoma. When followed over time, an increase in the white halo with diminution of the central nevus is commonly seen. Since a circumferential white halo is very rarely seen in melanoma (0.4%), and when present other specific dermoscopic features for melanoma may be visualized, a confident diagnosis of halo nevi as benign is usually easily made.[10]

Recurrent nevi

Pigmentation in a scar following removal of a melanocytic lesion can be due to a true recurrence of the lesion or reactive pigment changes without proliferation of melanocytes.[11] While there can be a morphological overlap between these under dermoscopic examination, the presence of globules or a heterogeneous pattern favor a true recurrence of the lesion.[11] The management of recurrent nevi, while depending upon the original pathology, can be assisted by short-term digital dermoscopy monitoring, with lack of change after 3 months leading to observation (see Chapter 8).

Acral lentiginous nevi

Nevi on volar sites (palms or soles) have a distinct morphology that differs from nevi on non-volar body sites. While a number of variations have been described, the basic element of acral nevi is the parallel furrow pattern with its histopathological correlation of nevus cells found in the crista profunda limitans, an epidermal rete ridge underlying the surface furrow (see Chapter 2).[12] Depending upon the anatomical site on the sole of the foot the parallel furrow pattern may remain intact (non-arch), show a lattice-like pattern (arch) or fibrillar-filamentous pattern (weight bearing surface).[13] The dermoscopic features of acral nevi are[12–16]:

- symmetry of pattern (majority)
- parallel furrow pattern (common)
- lattice-like pattern (some)
- fibrillar-fillamentous pattern (some)
- homogeneous pattern (some)
- globular pattern (some)
- reticular (network) pattern (some)
- globulostreak-like pattern (some)

Depending upon the series, 5–15% of acral nevi show non-typical patterns not described above.[12]

Dysplastic (Clark's) nevi

Dysplastic nevi are melanocytic nevi with cytologic atypia of junctional melanocyte/nevus cells in association with architectural atypia. Melanoma arises from dysplastic nevi more frequently than from common nevi. However, while they can be considered as an intermediate in the spectrum of common benign nevi and melanoma, they are benign. Because of their atypia, they possess greater morphological variability than any other benign pigmented lesion.[1,2,17] The major features of dysplastic nevi are:

- asymmetric pigmentation pattern (common)
- irregularly distributed and shaped brown globules (common)
- network irregular/discrete (common)
- network irregular/prominent (some)
- network edge abrupt (some)
- irregular/graduated edge (common)
- central black dots (some)
- irregular depigmentation (some)

MELANOCYTIC NEVI

Common benign acquired nevi (moles)

These lesions are formed from proliferating cells derived from melanocytes (nevus cells). They are categorized by the position of these cells in the skin. In general, the dermoscopy global patterns of these banal acquired nevi show a symmetrical pattern involving any of the three basic elements: network, globules, and homogeneous pigmentation.[1–2] The proportion of these elements differ with nevus type (junctional, compound, or dermal as detailed below) and age.

Globular patterns are more frequent in childhood and network (reticular) patterns more frequent in adults.[3] In skin type 1 individuals (who never tan following sun exposure), nevi are predominantly light brown in color, often with central hypopigmentation, whereas dark brown nevi become increasingly common as skin type increases (easier ability to tan). In skin type IV individuals (rarely burns) nevi with central increased pigmentation are common.[4] Finally, within individuals, repeated global patterns of nevi are often seen.[5,6]

Junctional nevi

Junctional nevi are composed of nests of nevus cells at the dermoepidermal junction. They are discrete, flat, pigmented lesions that have the dermoscopic features of:
- relatively regular/discrete network (majority)
- graduated regular edge (common)
- symmetrical pigmentation pattern (common)
- black dots/globules (uncommon or rarely seen)

Compound nevi

Compound nevi have nevus cells both at the dermoepidermal junction and in the dermis. They have the dermoscopic features of:
- areas of regular/discrete network (common)
- areas of uniform homogeneous pigmentation (common)
- graduated edge (common)
- symmetrical pigmentation pattern (common)
- regular depigmentation, often central (common)
- brown globules, uniform in shape and size (common)

Whether a compound nevus has a majority of its lesion containing a network, rather than areas of homogeneous pigmentation, depends on the relative amounts of junctional and dermal components (i.e. the network is formed by the junctional component and the homogeneous pigmentation by the dermal component). Indeed, it is not uncommon for compound nevi to lack the presence of a network when the junctional component is sparse.

Dermal nevi

The dermal nevus is formed entirely by nevus cells in the dermis. Following a general principle of dermoscopy that *associates increasing depth of pathology in the skin with a decrease in morphological definition,* dermal nevi are relatively structureless. The features of dermal nevi are:
- absent network, brown and black dots/globules (universal)
- faint homogeneous pigmentation (common)
- comma vessels (common)
- amelanotic (some)
- papillomatous cobblestone pattern (some)

While dermal nevi can contain telangiectases, they are generally less vascular than amelanotic nodules of invasive melanoma and nodular BCCs. Comma vessels, preferentially found at the periphery, are the most frequently found telangiectasia in dermal nevi.

Congenital nevi

Congenital melanocytic nevi are present at birth and are classified by their size: small (<1.5 cm diameter), intermediate (1.5–20 cm) or large (>20 cm). Under dermoscopy examination they tend to have more structures than benign non-congenital acquired nevi.[7] Furthermore, they have the

following features more frequently seen than non-congenital benign nevi: globular pattern, increased number of hair follicles, loss of pigment in the skin furrows, focal broadening of the network, target network, target globules, and vascular structures.[7] The dermoscopic features of congenital nevi are:[7–9]

- pigment network (common)
- globules (common)
- homogeneous pigmentation (common)
- hair follicles (often with surrounding depigmentation) (common)
- milia-like cysts (common)
- skin furrow hypopigmentation (common)
- vessels (common)
- target globules (some)
- target network (some)
- focal broadened network (some)

Like all nevi, loss of pigment around the hair follicles (perifollicular depigmentation) can be seen. Finally, both age and site can influence the dermoscopic appearance of congenital nevi, with globular patterns more frequent in childhood and reticular patterns preferentially seen on the limbs.[7,8]

Halo nevi

Halo nevi present as peripherally regressing benign nevi most commonly seen in adolescence and preferentially on the trunk.[10] Under dermoscopy examination the central nevus most frequently has either a globular or homogeneous pigmentation pattern without specific features for melanoma. When followed over time, an increase in the white halo with diminution of the central nevus is commonly seen. Since a circumferential white halo is very rarely seen in melanoma (0.4%), and when present other specific dermoscopic features for melanoma may be visualized, a confident diagnosis of halo nevi as benign is usually easily made.[10]

Recurrent nevi

Pigmentation in a scar following removal of a melanocytic lesion can be due to a true recurrence of the lesion or reactive pigment changes without proliferation of melanocytes.[11] While there can be a morphological overlap between these under dermoscopic examination, the presence of globules or a heterogeneous pattern favor a true recurrence of the lesion.[11] The management of recurrent nevi, while depending upon the original pathology, can be assisted by short-term digital dermoscopy monitoring, with lack of change after 3 months leading to observation (see Chapter 8).

Acral lentiginous nevi

Nevi on volar sites (palms or soles) have a distinct morphology that differs from nevi on non-volar body sites. While a number of variations have been described, the basic element of acral nevi is the parallel furrow pattern with its histopathological correlation of nevus cells found in the crista profunda limitans, an epidermal rete ridge underlying the surface furrow (see Chapter 2).[12] Depending upon the anatomical site on the sole of the foot the parallel furrow pattern may remain intact (non-arch), show a lattice-like pattern (arch) or fibrillar-filamentous pattern (weight bearing surface).[13] The dermoscopic features of acral nevi are[12–16]:

- symmetry of pattern (majority)
- parallel furrow pattern (common)
- lattice-like pattern (some)
- fibrillar-fillamentous pattern (some)
- homogeneous pattern (some)
- globular pattern (some)
- reticular (network) pattern (some)
- globulostreak-like pattern (some)

Depending upon the series, 5–15% of acral nevi show non-typical patterns not described above.[12]

Dysplastic (Clark's) nevi

Dysplastic nevi are melanocytic nevi with cytologic atypia of junctional melanocyte/nevus cells in association with architectural atypia. Melanoma arises from dysplastic nevi more frequently than from common nevi. However, while they can be considered as an intermediate in the spectrum of common benign nevi and melanoma, they are benign. Because of their atypia, they possess greater morphological variability than any other benign pigmented lesion.[1,2,17] The major features of dysplastic nevi are:

- asymmetric pigmentation pattern (common)
- irregularly distributed and shaped brown globules (common)
- network irregular/discrete (common)
- network irregular/prominent (some)
- network edge abrupt (some)
- irregular/graduated edge (common)
- central black dots (some)
- irregular depigmentation (some)

- small focal areas of multiple blue-gray dots (some)
- absent pseudopods, radial streaming, blue-white veil and multiple brown dots

While multiple blue-gray dots is a significant feature of melanoma, dysplastic nevi can have small focal areas (<10% of the lesion surface area) of multiple blue-gray dots without other dermoscopic features of melanoma.[18,19] In such cases observation is only required. Because all dysplastic nevi have a junctional component, no distinction is made here between junctional and compound dysplastic nevi.

Global patterns have also been described in dysplastic nevi, such as those having a multifocal hyper- or hypopigmented pattern, eccentric hyperpigmentation, and multicomponent pattern (all three, network, globular, and homogeneous structures). However, if these nevi lack specific dermoscopic features of melanoma they can be considered benign.[20]

Pigmented Spitz nevi

This benign tumor, most commonly seen in childhood, can be clinically and historically confused with melanoma. The diagnosis is less difficult in the initially rapidly growing amelanotic nodular variant seen on the face in children. However, in the pigmented variant, distinguishing these lesions from melanoma can be difficult (particularly in the adult). The dermoscopic features are very variable in Spitz nevi. This probably reflects the fact that an individual Spitz nevus can undergo dramatic global dermoscopic changes over time.[21,22] However, dermoscopy improves the diagnosis of Spitz nevi, with their features[21-25] being:

- symmetrical pigmentation pattern (common)
- circumferential pseudopods or radial streaming in a "starburst" pattern (common)
- deep rim of peripheral brown globules (common)
- central retiform depigmentation (common)
- regular prominent network (some)
- dotted vessels (some)
- negative pigment network (some)
- coffee-bean-like appearance (some)
- regular distribution of black and brown dots/globules (some)

When lesions with dermoscopic features of Spitz nevi are asymmetric in pigmentation pattern, excision is warranted. Such asymmetry usually reflects histological atypia (atypical Spitz nevus) or melanoma.

Blue nevi

Blue nevi represent collections of benign melanocytes in the mid to lower dermis. Their dermoscopic features are[26]:

- homogeneous blue pigmentation (universal)
- homogeneous blue pigmentation throughout the entire lesion (common)
- absent network, brown and black dots/globules (near universal)
- areas of depigmentation (some)

Areas of depigmentation can be due to loss of melanin in nevus cells or sclerosis.

Combined nevi

The most common combined nevus is that showing the histological combination of a blue nevus and benign acquired nevus (compound or dermal).[27] Most frequently such nevi show a central homogeneous area of blue pigmentation with surrounding dermoscopic features of compound or dermal nevi. However, when asymmetrical in pigmentation pattern, these lesions can mimic invasive melanoma under dermoscopy examination.

References

The text is based on the authors' observations and the following references:

1. Pehamberger, H, Binder, M, Steiner, A, Wolff, K. In vivo epiluminescence microscopy: Improvement of early diagnosis of melanoma. *J Invest Dermatol* 1993; 100: 356S–62S.

2. Steiner, A, Binder, M, Schemper, M, et al. Statistical evaluation of epiluminescence microscopy criteria for melanocytic pigment skin lesions. *J Am Acad Dermatol* 1993; 29: 581–8.

3. Zalaudek, I, Grinschgl, S, Argenziano, G, et al. Age-related prevalence of dermoscopy patterns in acquired melanocytic naevi. *Br J Dermatol* 2006; 154: 299–304.

4. Zalaudek, I, Argenziano, G, Mordente, I. Nevus type in dermoscopy is related to skin type in white persons. *Arch Dermatol* 2007; 143: 351–6.

5. Hofmann-Wellenhof, R, et al. Dermoscopic classification of atypical melanocytic nevi (Clark nevi). *Arch Dermatol* 2001: 137: 1575–80.

6. Scope, A, Burroni, M, Agero, AL, Benvenuto-Andrade, C, et al. Predominant dermoscopic patterns observed among nevi. *J Cutan Med Surg* 2006; 10: 170–4.

7. Seidenari, S, Pellacani, G, Martella, A, Giusti, F. Instrument-, age- and site-dependent variations of dermoscopic patterns of congenital melanocytic naevi: a multicentre study. *Br J Dermatol* 2006; 155: 56–61.

8. Changchien, L, Dusza, SW, Agero, AL, et al. Age- and site-specific variation in the dermoscopic patterns of congenital melanocytic nevi: an aid to accurate classification and assessment of melanocytic nevi. *Arch Dermatol* 2007; 143: 1007–14.

9. Ingordo, V, Iannazzone, SS, Cusano, F, Naldi, L. Dermoscopic features of congenital melanocytic nevus and Becker nevus in an adult male population: an analysis with a 10-fold magnification. *Dermatology* 2006; 212: 354–60.

10. Kolm, I, Di Stefani, A, Hofmann-Wellenhof, R, et al. Dermoscopy patterns of halo nevi. *Arch Dermatol* 2006; 142: 1627–32.

11. Botella-Estrada, R, Nagore, E, Sopena, et al. Clinical, dermoscopy and histological correlation study of melanotic pigmentations in excision scars of melanocytic tumours. *Br J Dermatol* 2006; 154: 478–84.

12. Saida, T, Koga, H. Dermoscopic patterns of acral melanocytic nevi: their variations, changes, and significance. *Arch Dermatol* 2007; 143: 1423–6.

13. Miyazaki, A, Saida, T, Koga, H, Oguchi, S, Suzuki, T, Tsuchida, T. Anatomical and histopathological correlates of the dermoscopic patterns seen in melanocytic nevi on the sole: a retrospective study. *J Am Acad Dermatol* 2005; 53: 230–6.

14. Ozdemir, F, Karaarslan, IK, Akalin, T. Variations in the dermoscopic features of acquired acral melanocytic nevi. *Arch Dermatol* 2007; 143: 1378–84.

15. Altamura, D, Altobelli, E, Micantonio, T, Piccolo, D, Fargnoli, MC, Peris, K. Dermoscopic patterns of acral melanocytic nevi and melanomas in a white population in central Italy. *Arch Dermatol* 2006; 142: 1123–8.

16. Malvehy, J, Puig, S. Dermoscopic patterns of benign volar melanocytic lesions in patients with atypical mole syndrome. *Arch Dermatol* 2004; 140: 538–44.

17. Carli, P, De Giorgi, V, Massi, D, Giannotti, B. The role of pattern analysis and the ABCD rule of dermoscopy in the detection of histological atypia in melanocytic naevi. *Br J Dermatol* 2000; 143: 290–7.

18. Zalaudek, I, Argenziano, G, Ferrara, G, et al. Clinically equivocal melanocytic skin lesions with features of regression: a dermoscopic-pathological study. *Br J Dermatol* 2004; 150: 64–71.

19. Braun, RP, Gaide, O, Oliviero, M, Kopf, AW, French, LE, Saurat, JH, Rabinovitz, HS. The significance of multiple blue-grey dots (granularity) for the dermoscopic diagnosis of melanoma. *Br J Dermatol* 2007; 157: 907–13.

20. Arevalo, A, Altamura, D, Avramidis, M, Blum, A, Menzies, SW. The significance of eccentric and central hyperpigmentation, multifocal hyper-hypopigmentation and the multicomponent pattern in melanocytic lesions lacking specific dermoscopy features of melanoma. *Arch Dermatol* 2008; 144: 1440–4.

21. Pizzichetta, MA, Argenziano, G, Grandi, G, de Giacomi, C, Trevisan, G, Soyer, HP. Morphologic changes of a pigmented Spitz nevus assessed by dermoscopy. *J Am Acad Dermatol* 2002; 47: 137–9.

22. Argenziano, G, Zalaudek, I, Ferrara, G, Lorenzoni, A, Soyer, HP. Involution: the natural evolution of pigmented Spitz and Reed nevi? *Arch Dermatol* 2007; 143: 549–5.

23. Steiner, A, Pehamberger, H, Binder, M, Wolff, K. Pigmented Spitz nevi: improvement of the diagnostic accuracy by epiluminescence microscopy. *J Am Acad Dermatol* 1992; 27: 697–701.

24. Ferrara, G, Argenziano, G, Soyer, HP, Chimenti, S, et al. The spectrum of Spitz nevi: a clinicopathologic study of 83 cases. *Arch Dermatol* 2005; 141: 1381–7.

25. Argenziano, G, Soyer, HP, Ferrara, G, Piccolo, D, et al. Superficial black network: an additional dermoscopic clue for the diagnosis of pigmented spindle and/or epithelioid cell nevus. *Dermatology* 2001; 203: 333–5.

26. Ferrara, G, Soyer, HP, Malvehy, J, Piccolo, D, Puig S, et al. The many faces of blue nevus: a clinicopathologic study. *J Cutan Pathol* 2007; 34: 543–51.

27. de Giorgi, V, Massi, D, Salvini, C, Trez, E, Mannone F, Carli P. Dermoscopic features of combined melanocytic nevi. *J Cutan Pathol* 2004; 31: 600–4.

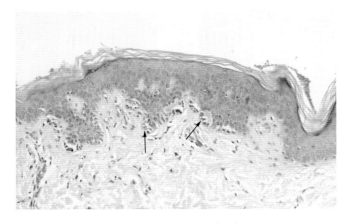

FIGURE 4.1 Junctional nevus (histopathology)
The junctional nevus shows nests of melanocytes at the dermoepidermal junction (arrow). There is also an increase in single melanocytes in the basal layer. In addition, the keratinocytes show increased pigmentation. Magnification ×50 (H & E stain).

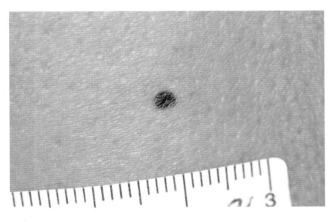

FIGURE 4.2 (a) Junctional nevus (clinical view)
Junctional nevi appear as discrete, usually flat (macular) pigmented lesions.

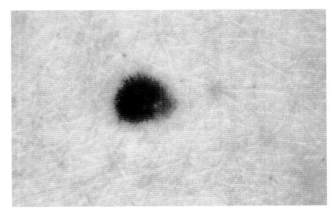

FIGURE 4.2 (b) Junctional nevus (dermoscopy)
The hall-mark of the junctional nevus is a relatively regular pigmented network.

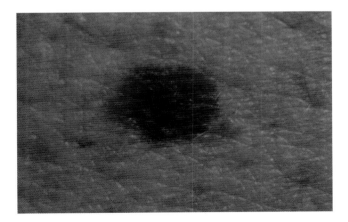

FIGURE 4.3 (a) Junctional nevus (clinical)

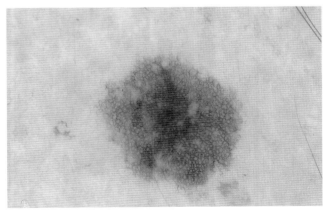

FIGURE 4.3 (b) Junctional nevus (dermoscopy)
The majority of banal acquired junctional nevi have a symmetrical network pattern throughout the lesion. These "reticular" nevi are more frequently found in adults.

FIGURE 4.4 Junctional nevus (dermoscopy)

The pigment network of junctional nevi tend to graduate at the edge. Black and brown dots/globules are uncommonly seen and when present usually only a few are found.

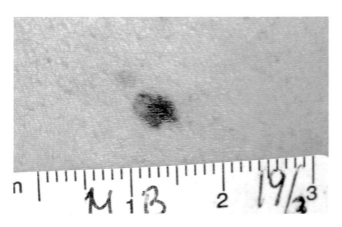

FIGURE 4.5 (a) Junctional nevus (clinical view)

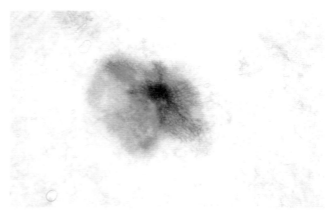

FIGURE 4.5 (b) Junctional nevus (dermoscopy)

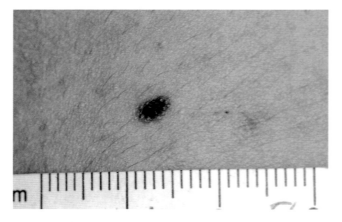

FIGURE 4.6 (a) Junctional nevus (clinical view)

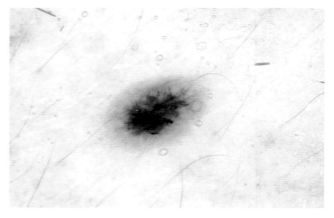

FIGURE 4.6 (b) Junctional nevus (dermoscopy)

While a few central black globules are present in this lesion, the network is regular and discrete (lightly pigmented) and graduated at the edge.

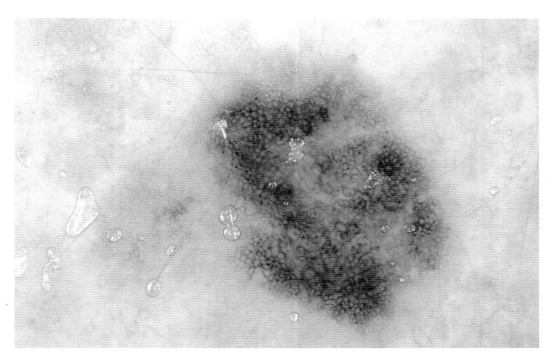

FIGURE 4.7 Junctional nevus (dermoscopy)
Note the brown dots/globules seen on the grids (cords) of the network. These represent nests of nevus cells at the tips of the rete ridges.

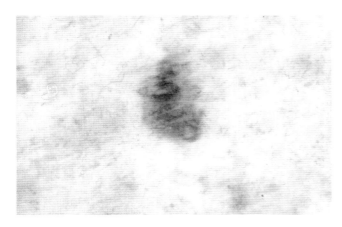

FIGURE 4.8 Junctional nevus (dermoscopy)
The pattern of the pigmented network can alter with different anatomical sites.

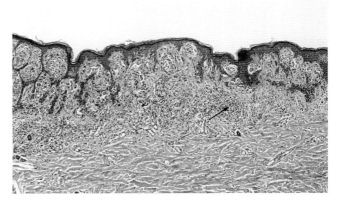

FIGURE 4.9 Compound nevus (histopathology)
The dermoepidermal junction shows nesting of melanocytes (similar to a junctional nevus). In addition there are melanocytes in the dermis (arrow). The melanocytes in nevi are called nevus cells or nevomelanocytes. Nevus cells are usually small, round or oval cells with a small nucleus and pale cytoplasm. The nucleus is larger than that of normal melanocytes found in the basal layer of the epidermis. Nevus cells may or may not contain pigment. Magnification ×16 (H & E stain).

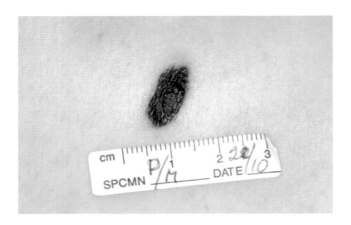

FIGURE 4.10 (a) Compound nevus (clinical view)

Compound nevi are discrete, usually raised and symmetrically pigmented lesions.

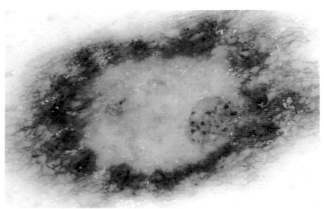

FIGURE 4.10 (b) Compound nevus (dermoscopy)

The junctional component of this compound nevus is seen as a discrete/ regular network surrounding its central dermal component (seen as regular homogeneous depigmentation). Brown globules are of regular distribution. Benign acquired nevi usually have one or more of three basic elements: network, dots/globules and homogeneous pigmentation. This lesion has all three, displaying the so called "multicomponent pattern". Multicomponent nevi that have no specific dermoscopic features of melanoma are benign.

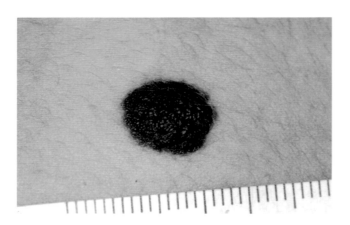

FIGURE 4.11 (a) Compound nevus (clinical view)

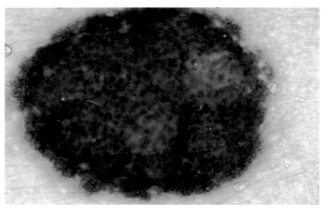

FIGURE 4.11 (b) Compound nevus (dermoscopy)

A common, unifying feature of benign nevi is a symmetrical pigmentation pattern.

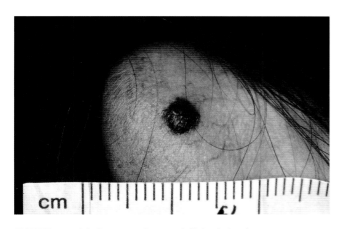

FIGURE 4.12 (a) Compound nevus (clinical view)

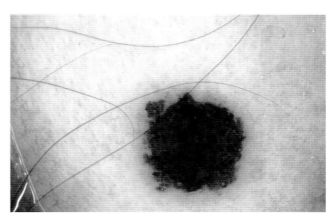

FIGURE 4.12 (b) Compound nevus (dermoscopy)

In this clinically suspicious lesion dermoscopy shows symmetrical pattern indicating its benign pathology. It should be noted (as seen here) that not all compound nevi have a pigment network.

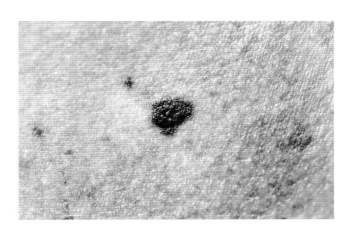

FIGURE 4.13 (a) Compound nevus (clinical view)

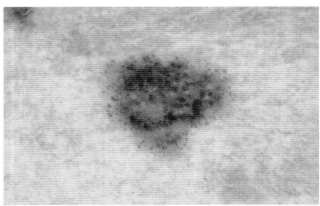

FIGURE 4.13 (b) Compound nevus—multiple peripheral brown globules (dermoscopy)

This variant of a compound nevus shows the presence of multiple peripheral brown globules. This type of nevus often has a relatively rapid radial growth, but is benign. Note the symmetrical pigmentation pattern. In some of these lesions the peripheral globules can form pseudopod-like structures. However, the diagnosis of pseudopods cannot be made in the presence of these globules.

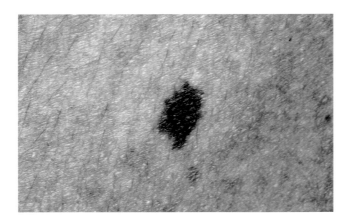

FIGURE 4.14 (a) Compound nevus (clinical view)

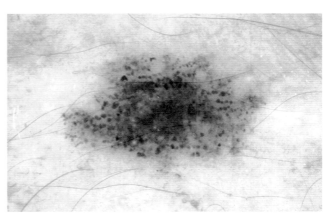

FIGURE 4.14 (b) Compound nevus (dermoscopy)
In this lesion the brown globules are again regular in distribution, with the lesion retaining symmetrical pigmentation pattern. Nevi with a globular pattern are more frequently found in childhood.

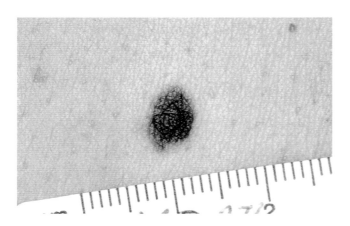

FIGURE 4.15 (a) Compound nevus (clinical view)

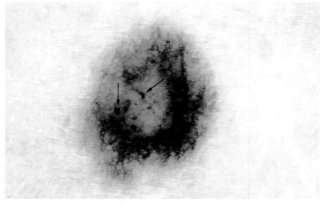

FIGURE 4.15 (b) Compound nevus (dermoscopy)
In some nevi of long standing, particularly congenital nevi, irregular crypts (arrow) and milia-like cysts are seen. However, in this case, no confusion exists with the differential diagnosis of a seborrheic keratosis because of the presence of an obvious, graduated pigment network. Seborrheic keratoses lack a pigment network.

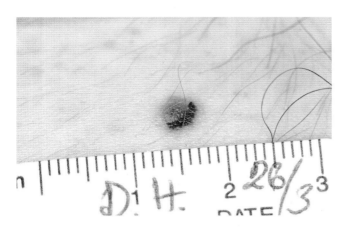

FIGURE 4.16 (a) Compound nevus (clinical view)

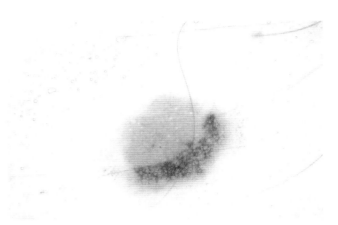

FIGURE 4.16 (b) Compound nevus (dermoscopy)
Note the multiple milia-like cysts but the obvious regular/discrete network that excludes the diagnosis of a seborrheic keratosis. This nevus has eccentric hyperpigmentation (a dark focus at the edge of the lesion). In the absence of specific dermoscopic features of melanoma (as seen here), such nevi are benign.

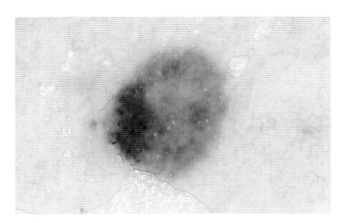

FIGURE 4.17 Compound nevus (dermoscopy)
Again this lesion shows eccentric hyperpigmentation. The absence of specific features of melanoma excludes the need for excision. Note the multiple small milia-like cysts in the central dermal component.

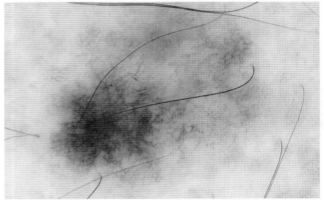

FIGURE 4.18 Compound nevus (dermoscopy)
Again the lesion has eccentric hyperpigmentation without specific features of melanoma.

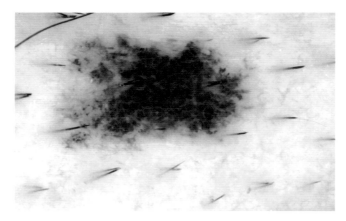

FIGURE 4.19 Compound nevus (dermoscopy)
A papillomatous cobblestone surface is seen in the dermal component of this lesion. Again, note the symmetrical pigmentation pattern.

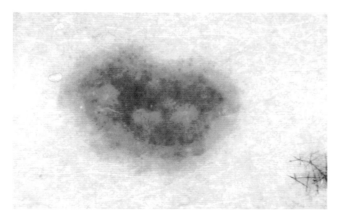

FIGURE 4.20 Compound nevus (dermoscopy)
Note the areas of uniform homogeneous pigmentation and lack of pigment network in this common presentation of a compound nevus. The relative amount of junctional versus dermal component determines whether a compound nevus has a majority of its area with a network compared with areas of homogeneous pigmentation (i.e. the network is formed from the junctional component and the homogeneous pigmentation from the dermal component). In this case, where the junctional component is sparse, no network is seen.

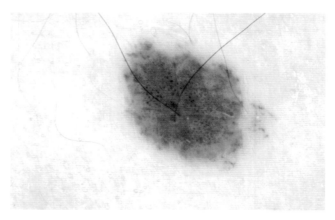

FIGURE 4.21 Compound nevus (dermoscopy)
A regular distribution of blue pigmentation is commonly seen in compound nevi. Note the regular distribution of brown globules.

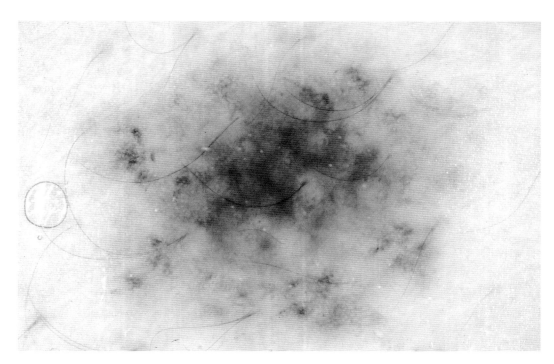

FIGURE 4.22 Compound nevus (dermoscopy)
Again, this lesion retains symmetrical pigmentation and has areas of regular/discrete network.

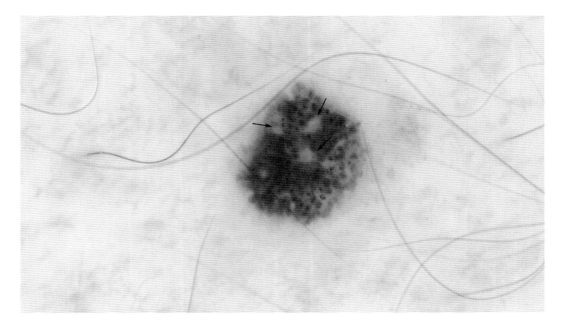

FIGURE 4.23 Compound nevus (dermoscopy)
This lesion has a globular pattern. Note the perifollicular depigmentation (arrows) which is commonly seen in nevi, particularly of the congenital variety.

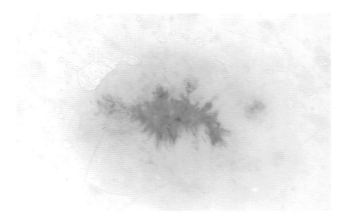

FIGURE 4.24 Compound nevus (dermoscopy)
Central stellate pigmentation in a near symmetrical pattern can be seen, albeit infrequently, in compound nevi.

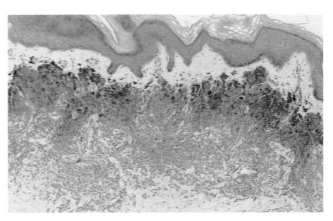

FIGURE 4.25 Dermal nevus (histopathology)
There is no junctional component in dermal nevi. Nevus cells are present only in the dermis. In this case the superficial nevus cells are pigmented. Magnification ×25 (H & E stain).

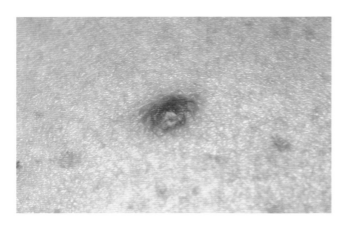

FIGURE 4.26 (a) Dermal nevus (clinical view)
Many dermal nevi, such as this lesion, are relatively amelanotic papules.

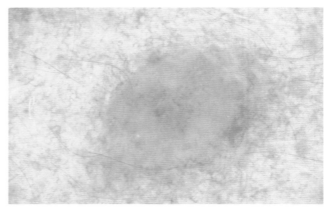

FIGURE 4.26 (b) Dermal nevus (dermoscopy)
Following a general principle of dermoscopy that associates increasing depth of pathology in the skin with a decrease in morphological definition, dermal nevi are often relatively structureless. This lesion has an hypomelanotic and avascular structure that is commonly seen with dermal nevi.

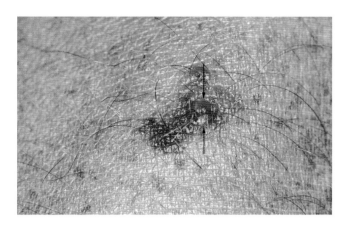

FIGURE 4.27 (a) Dermal nevus (clinical view)
The dermal component of this compound nevus is outlined by the arrows.

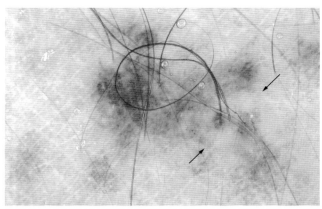

FIGURE 4.27 (b) Dermal nevus (dermoscopy)
Note that the corresponding area is relatively featureless. Often the dermal component of a nevus is "invisible" under dermoscopy.

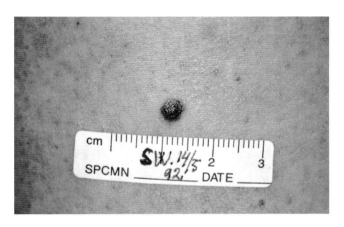

FIGURE 4.28 (a) Dermal nevus (clinical view)

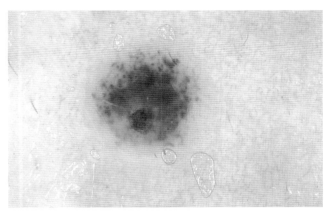

FIGURE 4.28 (b) Dermal nevus (dermoscopy)
All true dermal nevi lack a pigment network and black globules. Note the small erosion on the lesion's surface.

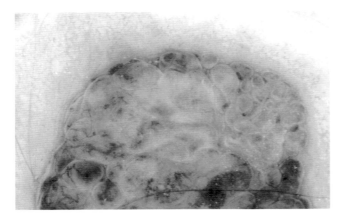

FIGURE 4.29 Dermal nevus (dermoscopy)
Many dermal nevi have a papillomatous surface. While vessels are found in some dermal nevi they are usually found in a preferentially peripheral position.

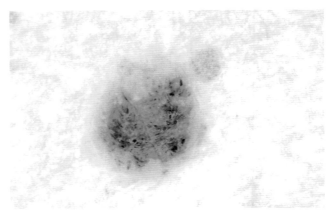

FIGURE 4.31 Dermal nevus (dermoscopy)
Small brown crypts and white milia-like cysts are seen.

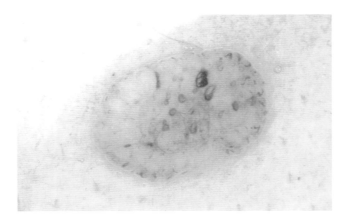

FIGURE 4.30 Dermal nevus (dermoscopy)
This dermal nevus has crypts present. Some dermal nevi are difficult to distinguish from seborrheic keratoses. Both lack a pigment network and may have milia-like cysts and crypts present. The soft consistency of this dermal nevus may differentiate it from a seborrheic keratosis. In addition, while telangiectases are present here, dermal nevi tend to be less vascular than amelanotic nodular melanomas. Here the predominant telangiectases present are comma vessels found in a predominantly peripheral position. The presence of regularly distributed comma vessels or comma vessels as the predominant vessel type is rarely found in melanoma.

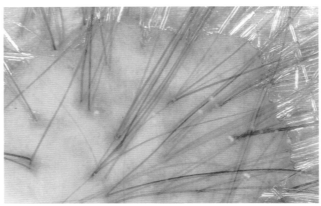

FIGURE 4.32 Dermal nevus (dermoscopy)

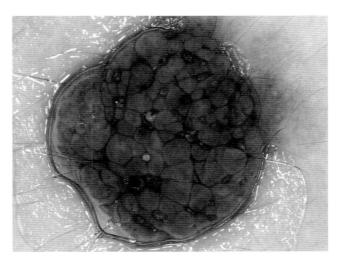

FIGURE 4.33 Dermal nevus (dermoscopy)
Again note the peripheral comma vessels and scattered crypts seen in some dermal nevi.

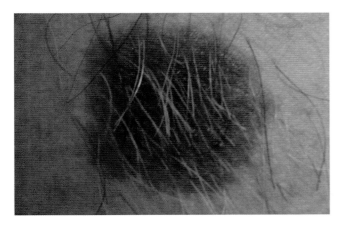

FIGURE 4.34 (a) Congenital nevus (clinical)

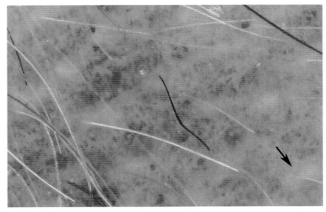

FIGURE 4.34 (b) Congenital nevus (dermoscopy)
Congenital nevi are more globular than non-congenital nevi. As well, hypertrichosis (increased hair follicles) often with depigmentation surrounding them are commonly seen (arrow).

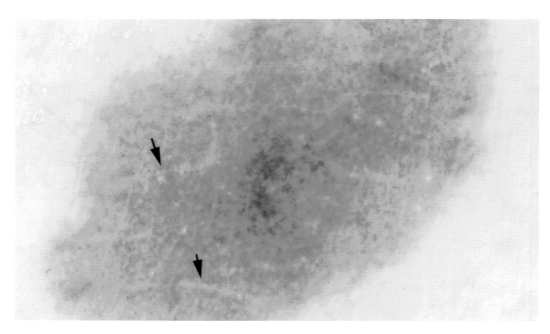

FIGURE 4.35 Congenital nevus (dermoscopy)
Congenital nevi are also characterized by an increase incidence of skin furrow hypopigmentation (arrows) and small milia-like cysts (seen here centrally).

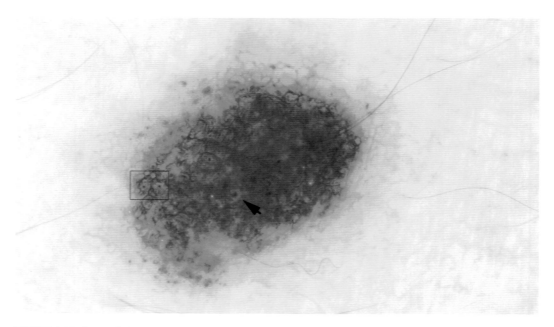

FIGURE 4.36 Congenital nevus (dermoscopy)
Here target globules are seen (globules with a white halo: arrow) in addition to a target network (target globules with a surrounding network: box). Both of these features are more frequently found in congenital compared with acquired nevi.

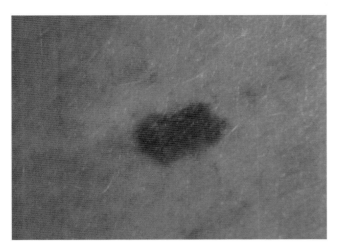

FIGURE 4.37 (a) Halo nevus (clinical)

Halo nevi present as peripherally regressing benign nevi most commonly seen in adolescence and preferentially on the trunk.

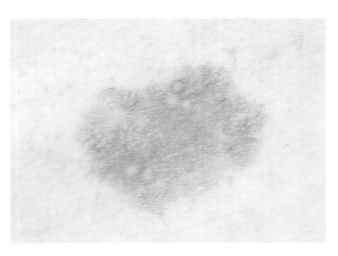

FIGURE 4.37 (b) Halo nevus (dermoscopy)

Under dermoscopy examination the central nevus lacks specific features for melanoma. Since a circumferential white halo is very rarely seen in melanoma (0.4%), and when a halo is present in melanoma other specific dermoscopic features for melanoma may be visualized, a confident diagnosis of halo nevi as benign is usually easily made.

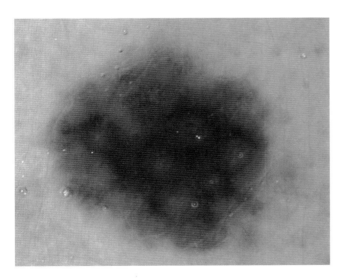

FIGURE 4.38 (a) Halo nevus (dermoscopy)*

This photograph was kindly provided by Dr Ignazio Stanganelli, Meldola-Forli, Italy.

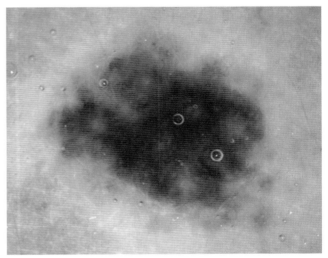

FIGURE 4.38 (b) Halo nevus (dermoscopy)†

This image was taken six months later. When followed in time, an increase in the white halo with diminution of the central nevus is commonly seen.

† This photograph was kindly provided by Dr Ignazio Stanganelli, Meldola-Forli, Italy.

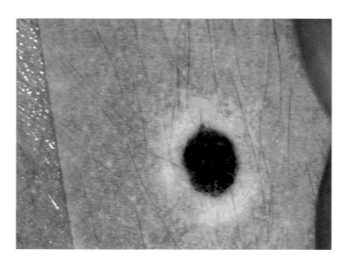

FIGURE 4.39 (a) Halo nevus (low magnification dermoscopy)‡
This image was taken on the trunk of a 16-year-old girl.

‡ *This photograph was kindly provided by Dr Ignazio Stanganelli, Meldola-Forli, Italy.*

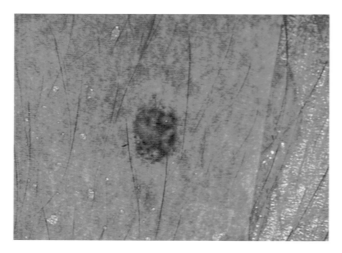

FIGURE 4.39 (b) Halo nevus (low magnification dermoscopy)§
The image was taken one year later.

§ *This photograph was kindly provided by Dr Ignazio Stanganelli, Meldola-Forli, Italy.*

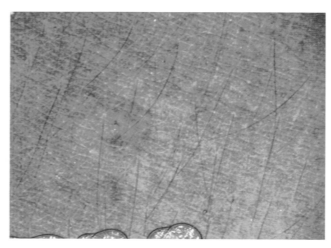

FIGURE 4.39 (c) Halo nevus (low magnification dermoscopy)¶
Complete resolution is seen three years from the baseline image.

¶ *This photograph was kindly provided by Dr Ignazio Stanganelli, Meldola-Forli, Italy.*

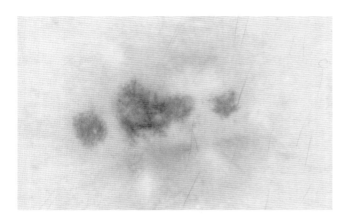

FIGURE 4.40 Recurrent nevus (dermoscopy)
Pigmentation in a scar following removal of a melanocytic lesion can be due to a true recurrence of the lesion or reactive pigment changes without proliferation of melanocytes. While there can be a morphological overlap between these under dermoscopic examination, the presence of globules or a heterogeneous pattern (both seen here) suggests a true recurrence of the lesion. If the original pathology showed only minor atypia and no dermoscopy evidence of melanoma is seen, short-term digital dermoscopy monitoring can aid in the management of such lesions.

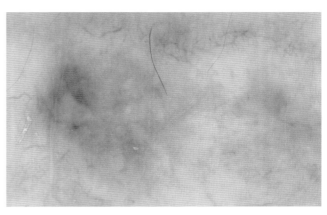

FIGURE 4.41 Reactive pigmentation in a scar (dermoscopy)
The homogeneous pattern confined within the scar favors reactive pigmentation (due to epidermal melanocytic hyperplasia or increased epidermal basal pigmentation without melanocytic proliferation) rather than a true recurrent lesion.

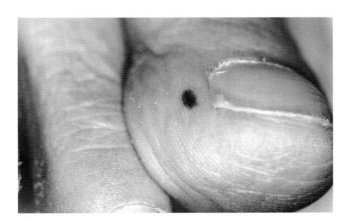

FIGURE 4.42 (a) Junctional nevus—acral lentiginous (clinical view)

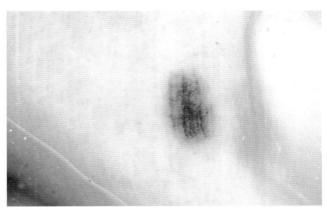

FIGURE 4.42 (b) Junctional nevus—acral lentiginous (dermoscopy)
The most common network pattern seen in benign volar (acral lentiginous) nevi is the parallel furrow pattern, where the parallel furrows of the surface skin markings are preferentially pigmented. When lines cross these furrows, as seen here, a lattice-like pattern is formed. The solitary finding of a lattice-like pattern confirms its benign diagnosis.

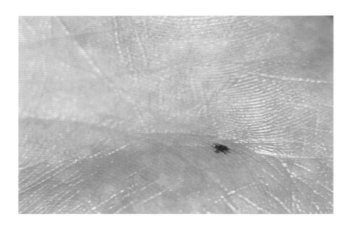

FIGURE 4.43 (a) Junctional nevus—acral lentiginous (clinical view)

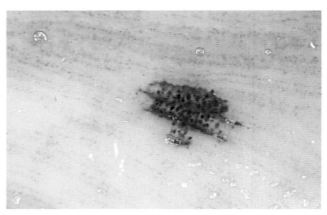

FIGURE 4.43 (b) Junctional nevus—acral lentiginous (dermoscopy)

This nevus on the palm has a variant of parallel furrow pattern with the addition of uniformly distributed brown globules.

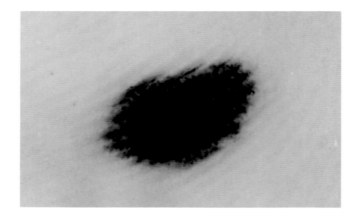

FIGURE 4.44 Junctional nevus—acral lentiginous (dermoscopy)

Again, this nevus has the parallel furrow pattern with the addition of uniformly distributed brown globules. On the sole of the foot the pattern depends upon the location of the nevus. Parallel furrow pattern preferentially occurs on the non-arch areas, lattice pattern on the arch and fibrillar filamentous pattern on the weight-bearing surface.

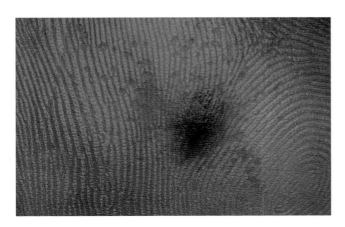

FIGURE 4.45 (a) Compound nevus—acral lentiginous (clinical view)

FIGURE 4.45 (b) Compound nevus—acral lentiginous (dermoscopy)

This compound nevus on the sole of foot has symmetrical pigmentation pattern and the fibrillar/filamentous pattern. Here a mesh-like or delicate filamentous pigmentation crossing the lines of skin markings is seen. While the blue pigmentation is somewhat unusual in these lesions (mimicking a combined nevus) the symmetry of pattern leads to a benign diagnosis.

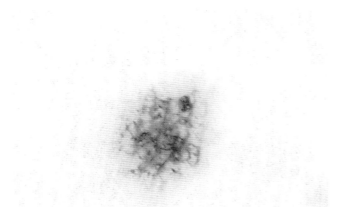

FIGURE 4.46 Compound nevus—acral lentiginous (dermoscopy)

This nevus on the sole has a somewhat irregular lattice-like pattern with pigmentation on the furrows and lines crossing the furrows.

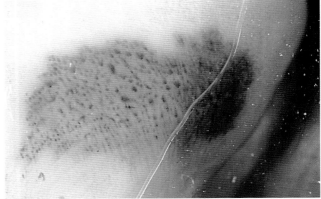

FIGURE 4.47 Compound nevus—acral lentiginous (dermoscopy)

Here the appearance of the pigmentation depends upon the orientation of the surface of the skin, with a globular pattern transforming into a fibrillar pattern.

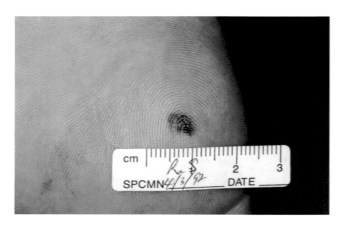

FIGURE 4.48 (a) Dermal nevus—acral lentiginous (clinical view)
Dermal nevi can appear relatively flat when present on the sole of the foot.

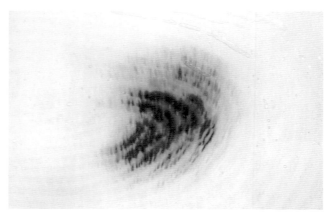

FIGURE 4.48 (b) Dermal nevus—acral lentiginous (dermoscopy)
This acral lentiginous dermal nevus on the sole of the foot has a fibrillar/ filamentous network pattern due to its position on the weight-bearing surface.

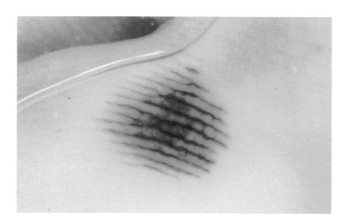

FIGURE 4.49 Nevus—acral lentiginous (dermoscopy)
The hallmark of benign nevi on volar sites is symmetry of pattern without the parallel ridge pattern (the parallel ridge pattern is found in 86% of melanoma and only 1% of nevi). Here the symmetrical parallel furrow pattern makes a benign diagnosis certain.

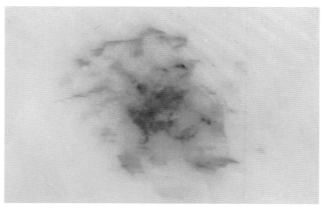

FIGURE 4.50 Nevus—acral lentiginous (dermoscopy)
Here a lattice pattern is seen with symmetry of pattern retained.

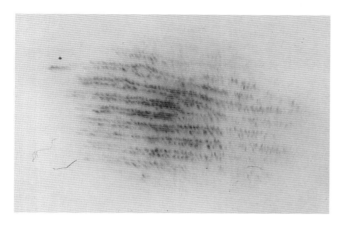

FIGURE 4.51 Nevus—acral lentiginous (dermoscopy)
The "train-track" variant of the parallel furrow pattern is seen.

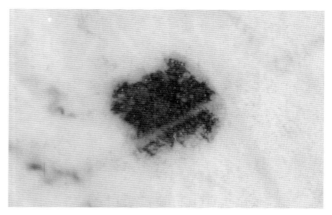

FIGURE 4.53 Nevus—acral lentiginous (dermoscopy)
This lesion has a reticular pattern mimicking nevi on non-volar sites.

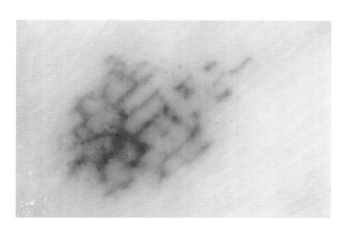

FIGURE 4.52 Nevus—acral lentiginous (dermoscopy)
Here the lattice pattern is seen.

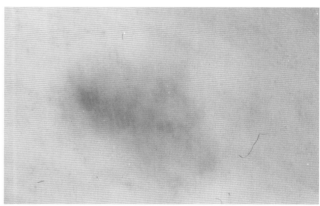

FIGURE 4.54 Nevus—acral lentiginous (dermoscopy)
This lesion has the homogeneous pattern.

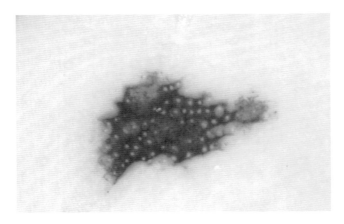

FIGURE 4.55 Nevus—acral lentiginous (dermoscopy)
Here the white eccrine (sweat) ducts are seen overlying the ridges. While the predominant pattern is lattice-like, disruption of the network forming small homogeneous areas of pigment lead to this nevus being digitally monitored.

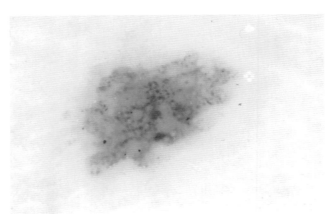

FIGURE 4.57 Nevus—acral lentiginous (dermoscopy)
This nevus has a non-typical pattern but lacks the two specific features of acral melanoma (parallel ridge pattern and irregular diffuse pigmentation with variable shades from tan to black: see Chapter 5) and is less than 7 mm in diameter. Such lesions can undergo digital monitoring to confirm a benign diagnosis (see Chapters 5 and 8).

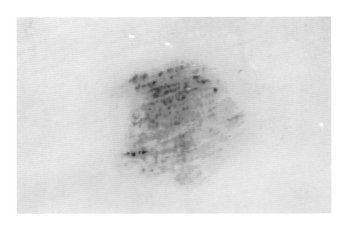

FIGURE 4.56 Nevus—acral lentiginous (dermoscopy)
Depending upon the series, 5–15% of acral nevi show non-typical patterns with mixed elements as seen here. Nevertheless the absence of parallel ridge pattern lead to this nevus being monitored rather than excised.

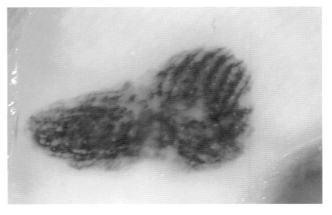

FIGURE 4.58 Nevus—acral lentiginous (dermoscopy)
When nevi cross the boundary of volar and non-volar skin the pigment network changes. Here the parallel furrow pattern is replaced by a more network like pattern simply due to differences in anatomical location. Such lesions should not be confused with non-typical patterns.

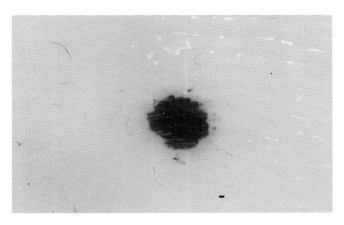

FIGURE 4.59 Subcorneal hemorrhage (dermoscopy)
A false parallel ridge pattern is seen in some subcorneal hemorrhages on volar surfaces.

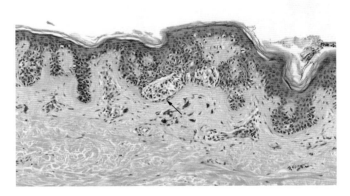

FIGURE 4.60 Dysplastic nevus (histopathology)
The concept and diagnosis of the dysplastic nevus is controversial. However, it is widely accepted that the histological diagnosis can be made in the appropriate clinical setting. The lesion should have architectural atypia such as bridging of nests of nevus cells across adjacent rete ridges (arrow) and cytological atypia of the nevus cells. Other features such as a lymphoid infiltrate and fibrosis in the superficial dermis are often present. Magnification ×50 (H & E stain).

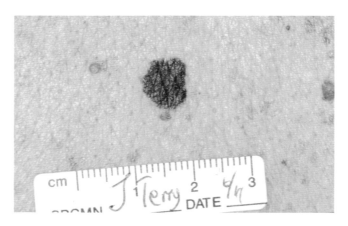

FIGURE 4.61 (a) Dysplastic nevus (clinical view)
Dysplastic nevi are seen as discrete, irregularly pigmented macules or papules. They are often larger than common nevi. Because all dysplastic nevi have a junctional component, no distinction is made here between junctional and compound dysplastic nevi.

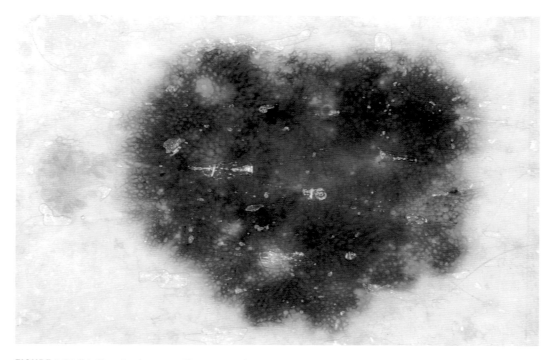

FIGURE 4.61 (b) Dysplastic nevus (dermoscopy)
This dysplastic nevus shows many of its common features, including asymmetric pigmentation pattern, areas of prominent (darkly pigmented) irregular network, central black dots/globules (compared with peripheral black dots/globules seen in melanoma) and an irregular/graduated edge. There are no pseudopods, radial streaming, blue-white veil and multiple brown dots (all highly specific for melanoma).

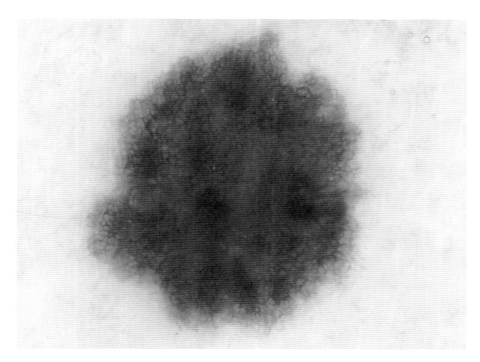

FIGURE 4.62 Dysplastic nevus (dermoscopy)
This characteristic presentation shows a lesion with an irregular prominent network without broadening
of the grids (cords) of the network.

FIGURE 4.63 Dysplastic nevus (dermoscopy)
Again typically, dysplastic nevi have asymmetry of pigmentation
pattern without any specific dermoscopic features of melanoma.

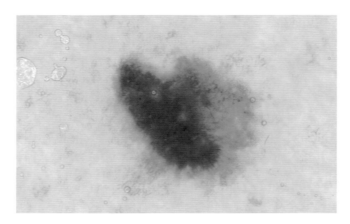

FIGURE 4.64 Dysplastic nevus (dermoscopy)

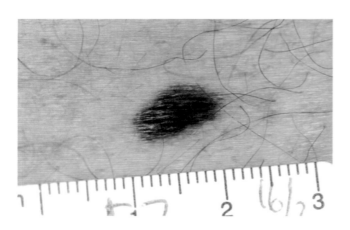

FIGURE 4.65 (a) Dysplastic nevus (clinical view)

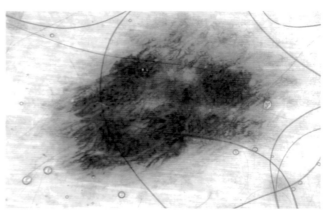

FIGURE 4.65 (b) Dysplastic nevus (dermoscopy)

Despite the clinically irregular nature of this lesion, under dermoscopy there are no features of melanoma. The network is discrete and graduated at the edge, with scattered irregular brown globules. In this lesion the lines of the network cause *false* radial streaming. Unlike true radial streaming, which appears confined to the edge as short radial projections, here the network forms areas of elongated strands that are also found within the lesion.

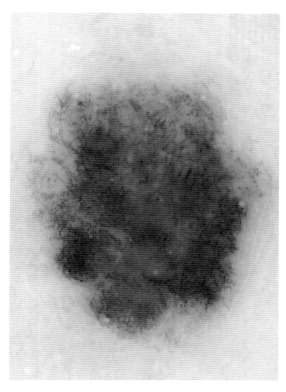

FIGURE 4.66 Dysplastic nevus (dermoscopy)
A common feature of dysplastic nevi is irregular depigmentation.

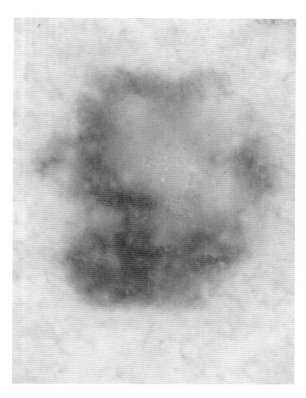

FIGURE 4.67 Dysplastic nevus (dermoscopy)
Again irregular depigmentation is seen here. In some cases this can be difficult to discern from scar-like depigmentation.

FIGURE 4.68 Dysplastic nevus (dermoscopy)

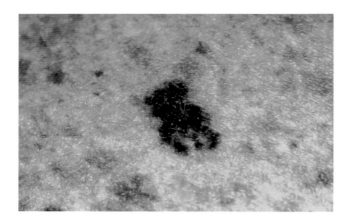

FIGURE 4.69 (a) Dysplastic nevus (clinical view)

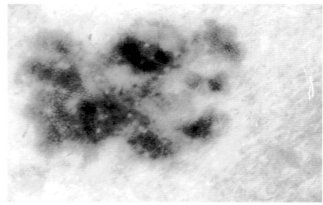

FIGURE 4.69 (b) Dysplastic nevus (dermoscopy)
While there is asymmetric pigmentation pattern in this lesion, no positive features of melanoma are seen.

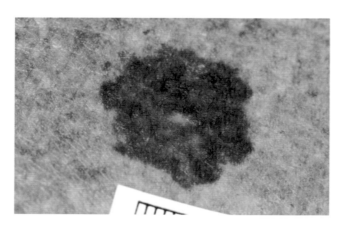

FIGURE 4.70 (a) Dysplastic nevus (clinical view)

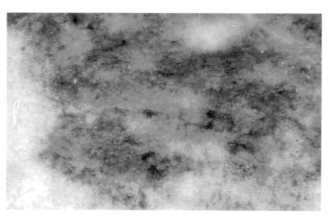

FIGURE 4.70 (b) Dysplastic nevus (dermoscopy)
In this representative section of the lesion, asymmetric pigmentation pattern consists of brown irregularly distributed globules, small areas of irregularly distributed blue pigment not forming blue-white veil, and areas of irregular/discrete network and central depigmentation.

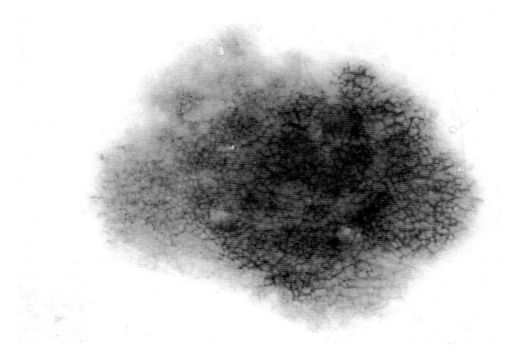

FIGURE 4.71 Dysplastic nevus (dermoscopy)
Note the areas of prominent (darkly pigmented) network, non-graduated (abrupt) edge of network, and central black dots/globules. In contrast to melanoma, the cords of the network are relatively uniform in thickness and not focally broadened.

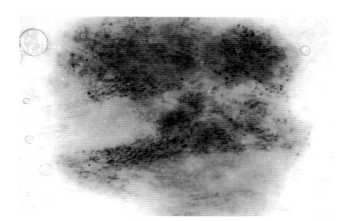

FIGURE 4.72 Dysplastic nevus (dermoscopy)
Note the areas of irregular depigmentation, irregularly distributed and shaped brown globules, and relatively central black globules.

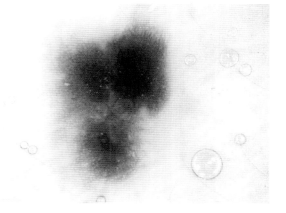

FIGURE 4.73 Dysplastic nevus (dermoscopy)
In this asymmetrically pigmented lesion no classic features of melanoma (pseudopods, radial streaming, blue-white veil, multiple brown dots, peripheral black dots/globules, multiple colors, multiple blue-gray dots, scar-like depigmentation and broadened network) are seen.

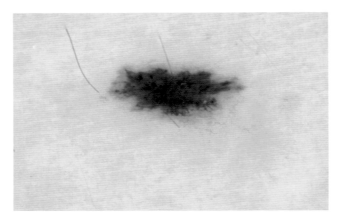

FIGURE 4.74 Dysplastic nevus (dermoscopy)
This lesion is characterized by symmetry of pattern and central black globules.

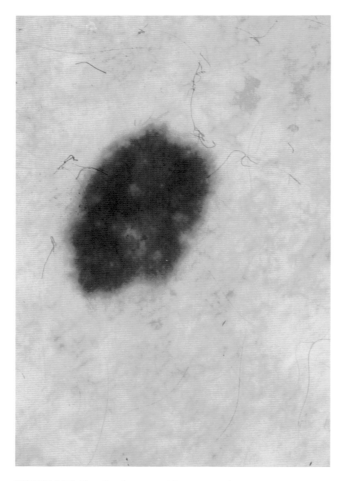

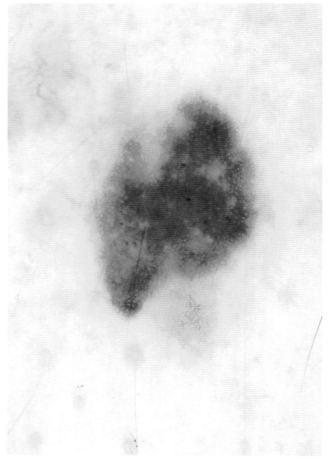

FIGURE 4.75 Dysplastic nevus (dermoscopy)
In this common presentation of dysplastic nevi confluent areas of blue pigmentation are seen relatively uniformly distributed within the lesion. Sometimes these areas can be difficult to distinguish from melanophages (multiple blue-gray dots). However, often a patient with such a nevus will have this pattern repeatedly seen in other nevi.

FIGURE 4.76 Dysplastic nevus (dermoscopy)

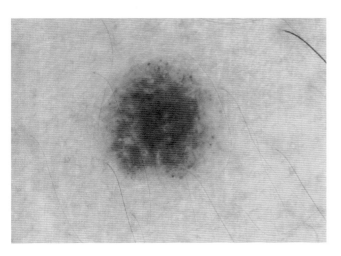

FIGURE 4.77 (a) Dysplastic nevus (dermoscopy)

As seen with benign acquired nevi, repeated patterns of dysplastic nevi in an individual patient can lead to a more confident diagnosis of a benign lesion. Here, all lesions seen in a–d belong to the same patient, with a repeated pattern of blue central pigmentation.

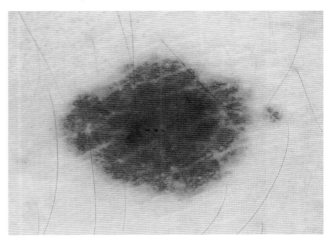

FIGURE 4.77 (c) Dysplastic nevus (dermoscopy)

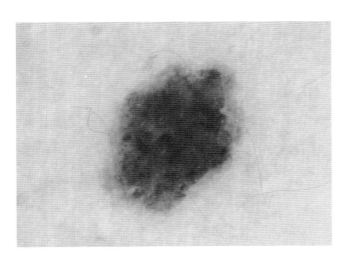

FIGURE 4.77 (b) Dysplastic nevus (dermoscopy)

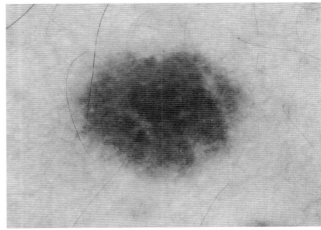

FIGURE 4.77 (d) Dysplastic nevus (dermoscopy)

FIGURE 4.78 Dysplastic nevus (dermoscopy)
Areas of negative pigment network are seen. While this feature is commonly seen in Spitz nevi and melanoma, it can also occur in dysplastic nevi.

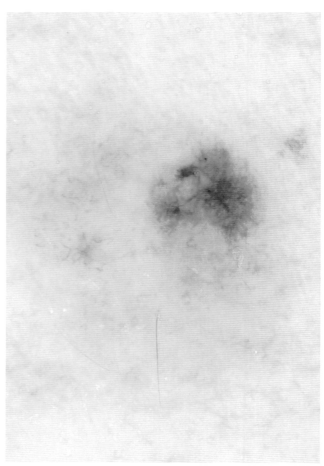

FIGURE 4.80 Dysplastic nevus (dermoscopy)
In this lesion with eccentric hyperpigmentation no dermoscopic features of melanoma can be seen. Hence observation is only required.

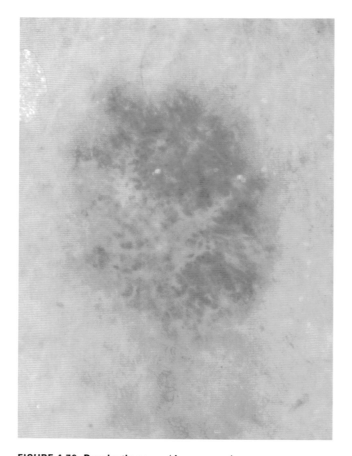

FIGURE 4.79 Dysplastic nevus (dermoscopy)
Again a widespread negative network is seen.

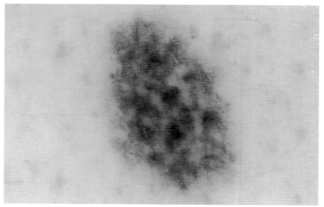

FIGURE 4.81 Dysplastic nevus (dermoscopy)
This lesion has the multifocal hyper/hypopigmentation pattern characteristic of some dysplastic nevi.

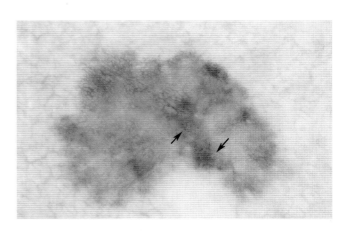

FIGURE 4.84 Dysplastic nevus (dermoscopy)
This lesion is characterized by irregular depigmentation and small areas of multiple blue-gray dots (arrows) occupying less than 10% of the surface area of the lesion.

FIGURE 4.82 Dysplastic nevus (dermoscopy)
Dysplastic nevi can present as pink lesions which are more difficult to be confident about the diagnosis (see Chapter 5 for details on distinguishing benign from malignant pink lesions).

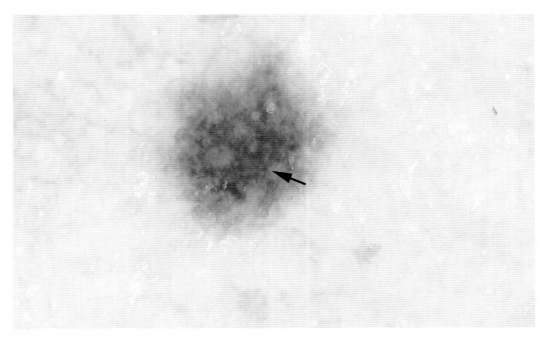

FIGURE 4.83 Dysplastic nevus (dermoscopy)
Small areas of multiple blue-gray dots (melanophages) can occur in dysplastic nevi (arrow). When found focally and occupying less than 10% of the surface area in a lesion without any other dermoscopy evidence of melanoma (as seen here), observation is only required.

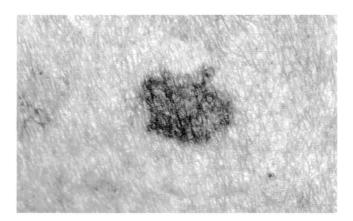

FIGURE 4.85 (a) Dysplastic nevus (clinical view)

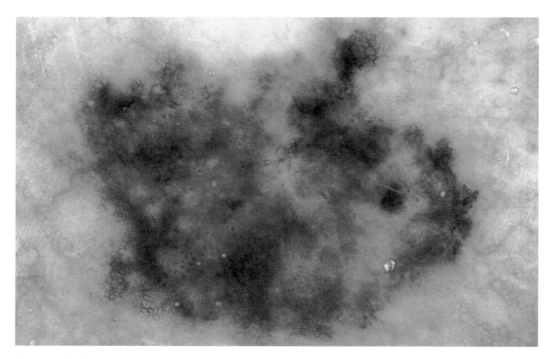

FIGURE 4.85 (b) Dysplastic nevus (dermoscopy)

Here numerous foci of multiple blue-gray dots are seen irregularly distributed throughout the lesion. Here excision is warranted to exclude melanoma.

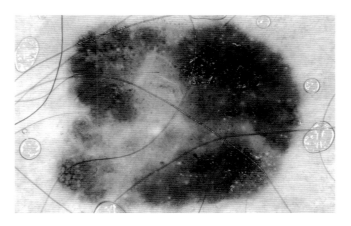

FIGURE 4.86 Dysplastic nevus (dermoscopy)
The main differential diagnosis of the dysplastic nevus is melanoma. Indeed, many dysplastic nevi have a specific dermoscopic feature of invasive melanoma and can only be confirmed as benign following histopathological examination. The observation of multiple colors, scar-like depigmentation and areas mimicking blue-white veil must lead to excision of this dysplastic nevus.

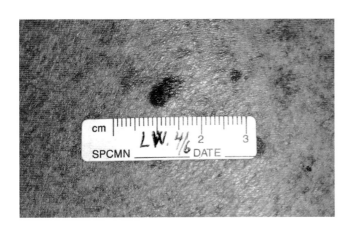

FIGURE 4.87 (a) Dysplastic nevus (clinical view)

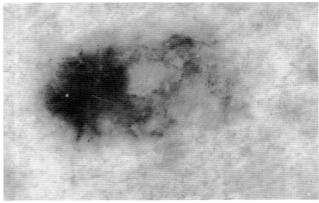

FIGURE 4.87 (b) Dysplastic nevus (dermoscopy)
While the observation of blue-white veil suggested the diagnosis of invasive melanoma, histopathological examination confirmed this lesion as a dysplastic nevus.

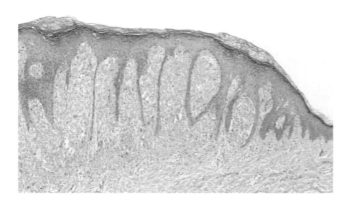

FIGURE 4.88 Spitz nevus (histopathology)

The Spitz nevus is usually a compound nevus composed of spindled and/ or epithelioid cells. While the Spitz nevus is benign, it may have some histological features resembling malignant melanoma. The cells may be large and pleomorphic and mitosis may be present. Differentiation from melanoma can be helped by the clinical information and features such as symmetry, maturation of the lesion (i.e. cells and their nuclei are smaller at the base of the lesion compared with the more superficial cells) and absence of mitoses deep within the lesion. Magnification ×16 (H & E stain).

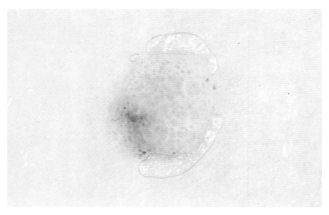

FIGURE 4.89 Spitz nevus (dermoscopy)

This benign tumor, most commonly seen in childhood, can be clinically confused with melanoma (hence the term "juvenile melanoma"). It may initially grow rapidly, with bleeding and crusting not uncommon. Here, the presence of a negative pigment network throughout the lesion leads to the diagnosis of Spitz nevus.

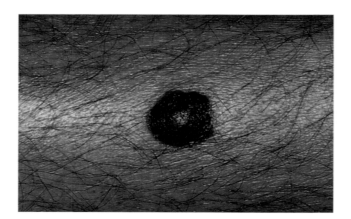

FIGURE 4.90 (a) Spitz nevus (clinical view)

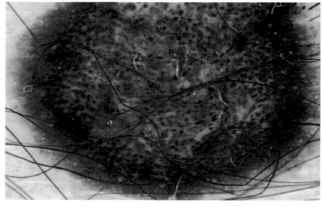

FIGURE 4.90 (b) Spitz nevus (dermoscopy)

One presentation of Spitz nevus is a central bizarre pattern of retiform depigmentation that tapers out, forming a negative pigment network. In this case, the regular repeated structure of the retiform depigmentation excludes the diagnosis of blue-white veil.

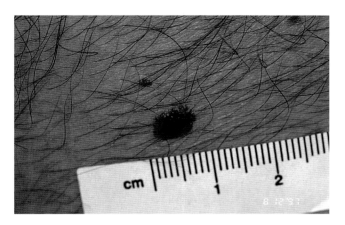

FIGURE 4.91 (a) Spitz nevus (clinical view)

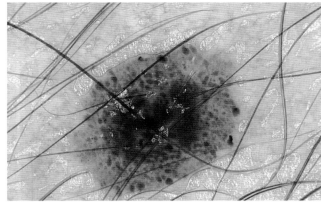

FIGURE 4.91 (b) Spitz nevus (dermoscopy)
A deep rim of peripheral brown globules can be seen in some Spitz nevi. Note also the symmetrical pigmentation pattern which is the hallmark of the majority of Spitz nevi.

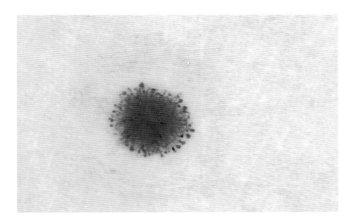

FIGURE 4.92 Spitz nevus (dermoscopy)
Some Spitz nevi have a uniform distribution of pseudopods around the edge of the lesion forming a "starburst" pattern. In melanoma, pseudopods are rarely if ever found in such a regular circumferential position. However, lesions with this morphology can be histopathologically difficult to distinguish from melanoma, as in this case.

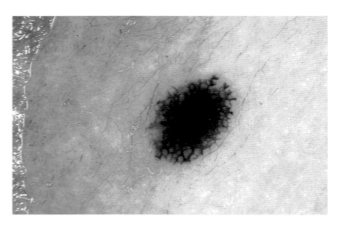

FIGURE 4.93 (a) Spitz nevus (clinical view)

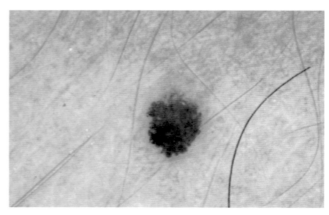

FIGURE 4.93 (b) Spitz nevus (dermoscopy)
This lesion has a prominent (dark) network characteristic of some Spitz nevi. Like dysplastic nevi, Spitz nevi are very morphologically variable. This morphological variability is in part due to the observation that an individual Spitz nevus can change its global pattern significantly over time.

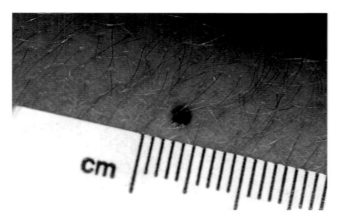

FIGURE 4.94 (a) Spitz nevus (clinical view)

FIGURE 4.94 (b) Spitz nevus (dermoscopy)

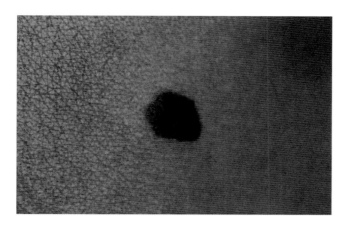

FIGURE 4.95 (a) Spitz nevus (clinical view)

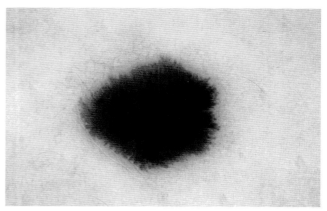

FIGURE 4.95 (b) Spitz nevus (dermoscopy)
In this lesion the starburst-like pattern is suggestive of a Spitz nevus. However, the asymmetric pigmentation pattern requires excision biopsy to confirm the diagnosis.

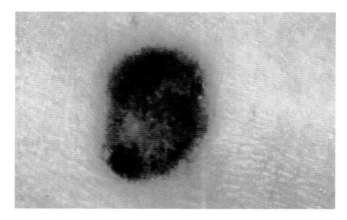

FIGURE 4.96 Spitz nevus (dermoscopy)
Central retiform depigmentation that tapers out, forming a negative pigment network, is seen here.

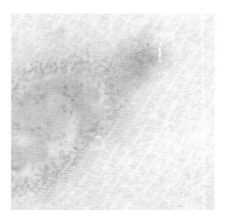

FIGURE 4.97 Spitz nevus (dermoscopy)
A deep rim of peripheral brown globules characterizes this Spitz nevus.

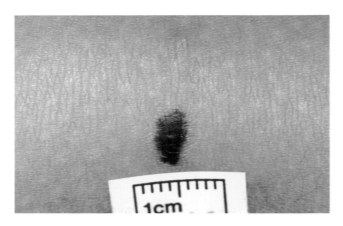

FIGURE 4.98 (a) Spitz nevus (spindle cell nevus of Reed) (clinical view)

In this variant of Spitz nevus (spindle cell nevus of Reed) the lesion appears characteristically ink-black.

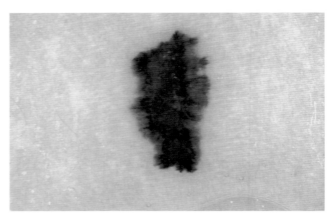

FIGURE 4.98 (b) Spitz nevus (spindle cell nevus of Reed) (dermoscopy)

This starburst-like pattern is formed from radial streaming-like extensions uniformly distributed throughout the lesion. Again, note the symmetrical pigmentation pattern.

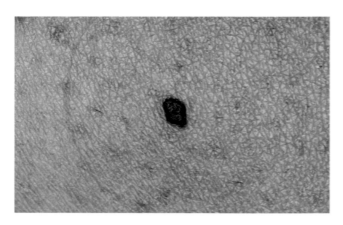

FIGURE 4.99 (a) Spitz nevus (spindle cell nevus of Reed) (clinical view)

In this classical presentation of a spindle cell nevus of Reed, this black lesion appeared suddenly on the thigh of a young woman. Clinically it is very difficult to exclude melanoma.

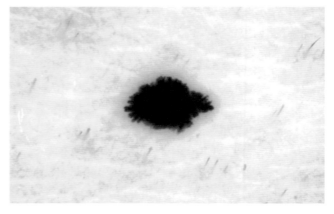

FIGURE 4.99 (b) Spitz nevus (spindle cell nevus of Reed) (dermoscopy)

The symmetry of pigmentation with a starburst pattern confirms the diagnosis.

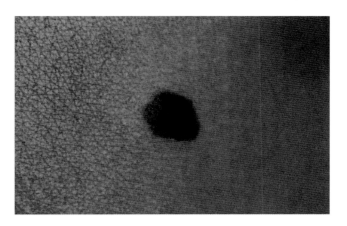

FIGURE 4.95 (a) Spitz nevus (clinical view)

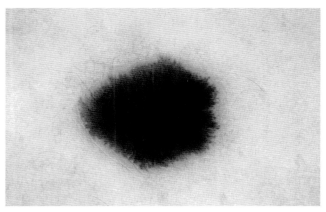

FIGURE 4.95 (b) Spitz nevus (dermoscopy)
In this lesion the starburst-like pattern is suggestive of a Spitz nevus. However, the asymmetric pigmentation pattern requires excision biopsy to confirm the diagnosis.

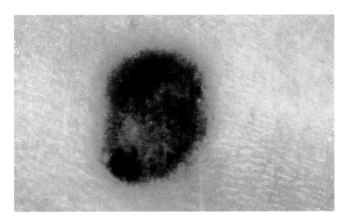

FIGURE 4.96 Spitz nevus (dermoscopy)
Central retiform depigmentation that tapers out, forming a negative pigment network, is seen here.

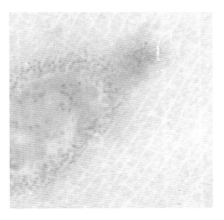

FIGURE 4.97 Spitz nevus (dermoscopy)
A deep rim of peripheral brown globules characterizes this Spitz nevus.

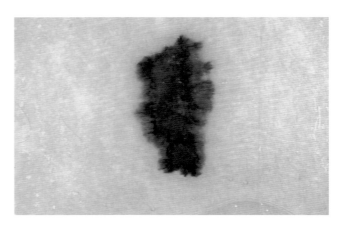

FIGURE 4.98 (a) Spitz nevus (spindle cell nevus of Reed) (clinical view)

In this variant of Spitz nevus (spindle cell nevus of Reed) the lesion appears characteristically ink-black.

FIGURE 4.98 (b) Spitz nevus (spindle cell nevus of Reed) (dermoscopy)

This starburst-like pattern is formed from radial streaming-like extensions uniformly distributed throughout the lesion. Again, note the symmetrical pigmentation pattern.

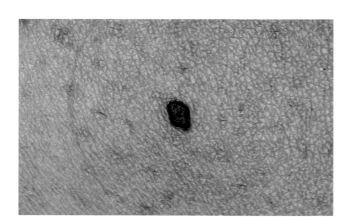

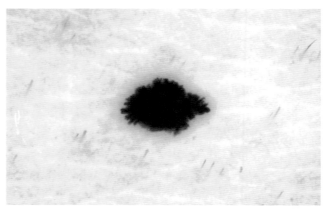

FIGURE 4.99 (a) Spitz nevus (spindle cell nevus of Reed) (clinical view)

In this classical presentation of a spindle cell nevus of Reed, this black lesion appeared suddenly on the thigh of a young woman. Clinically it is very difficult to exclude melanoma.

FIGURE 4.99 (b) Spitz nevus (spindle cell nevus of Reed) (dermoscopy)

The symmetry of pigmentation with a starburst pattern confirms the diagnosis.

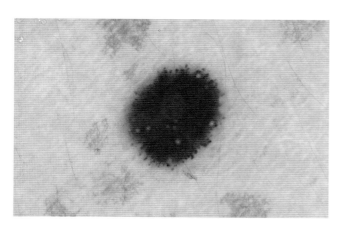

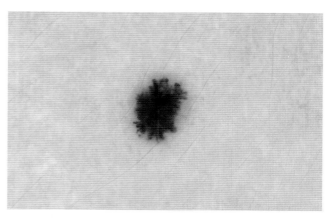

FIGURE 4.100 Spitz nevus (dermoscopy)
The rapid radial growth seen with some Spitz nevi, especially in the starburst or globular variants, makes the use of digital monitoring in their assessment more difficult than other nevi.

FIGURE 4.101 Spitz nevus (dermoscopy)
In this lesion, asymmetry of pattern and blue-white veil necessitates excision of the lesion.

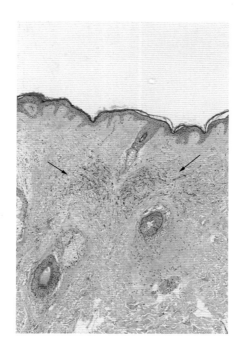

FIGURE 4.102 Blue nevus (histopathology)
In their most common form, blue nevi (delineated by arrows) show an intradermal, poorly circumscribed collection of elongated, pigmented melanocytes. The epidermis is not involved. The commonly seen grenz zone of absent melanocytes in the upper dermis is responsible for the solitary blue color seen under dermoscopy in the majority of blue nevi. Magnification ×16 (H & E stain).

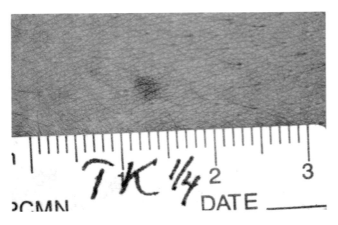

FIGURE 4.103 (a) Blue nevus (clinical view)

Blue nevi classically appear as uniformly blue pigmented macules or nodules.

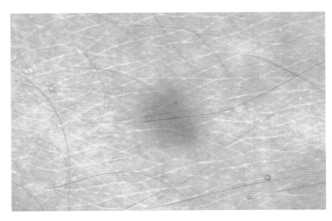

FIGURE 4.103 (b) Blue nevus (dermoscopy)

This lesion under dermoscopy shows the most common presenting morphology of blue nevi—a homogeneous blue pigmentation throughout the entire lesion.

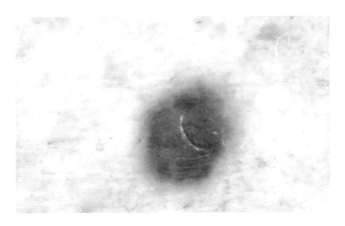

FIGURE 4.104 Blue nevus (dermoscopy)

No confusion should occur when excluding the melanoma-specific feature, blue-white veil, in this lesion. Blue-white veil is always seen as an irregular pattern that never occupies the entire lesion.

FIGURE 4.105 Blue nevus (dermoscopy)

In some blue nevi, areas of brown pigmentation are seen. However, a pigmented network and brown and black dots/globules are absent. It is this absence of features associated with an area mimicking blue-white veil that favors the diagnosis of blue nevus. However the differential diagnosis includes a combined nevus and melanoma.

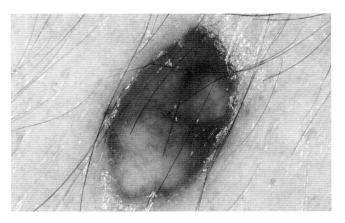

FIGURE 4.106 Blue nevus (dermoscopy)
In some blue nevi, areas of depigmentation can be seen. These may be due
to loss of melanin in the melanocytes or areas of sclerosis.

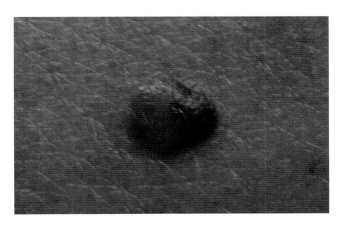

FIGURE 4.107 (a) Blue nevus (clinical)

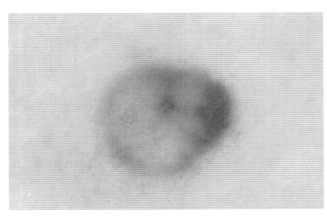

FIGURE 4.107 (b) Blue nevus (dermoscopy)
Here depigmentation is due to extensive sclerotic collagen bundles in the
superficial dermis.

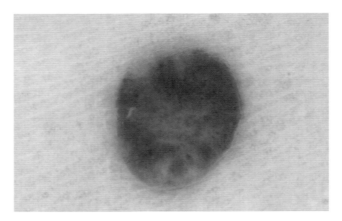

FIGURE 4.108 Blue nevus (dermoscopy)

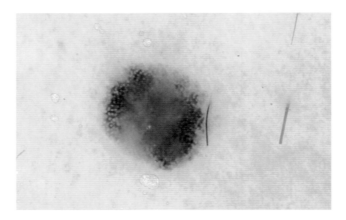

FIGURE 4.109 Blue nevus (dermoscopy)
This atypical presentation of a blue nevus shows a definite pigment network. However this network was due to increased basal pigmentation of the epidermis without melanocytic proliferation.

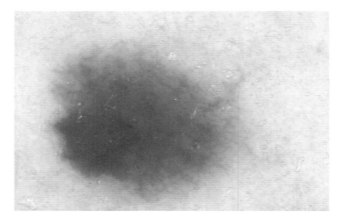

FIGURE 4.110 Blue nevus (dermoscopy)
Some blue nevi have blue network-like areas at their edge. This should be distinguished from a true pigmented network, which is always brown.

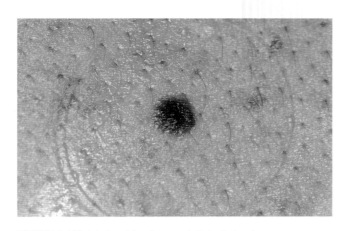

FIGURE 4.111 (a) Combined nevus (clinical view)

A blue nevus can be superimposed on a benign common nevus resulting in a "combined nevus".

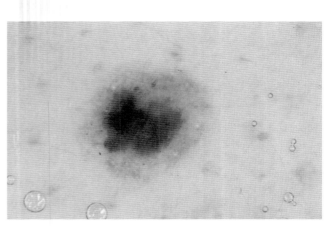

FIGURE 4.111 (b) Combined nevus (dermoscopy)

The central blue nevus is seen with a superimposed compound nevus. In this case, it may be difficult to decide between the diagnosis of a combined nevus and a melanoma arising from a nevus, since the blue nevus mimicks blue-white veil.

FIGURE 4.112 Combined nevus (dermoscopy)

In this more typical case, the central focus of uniform blue homogeneous pigmentation (blue nevus) surrounded by a uniform tan pigment (compound nevus) leads to the diagnosis of combined nevus.

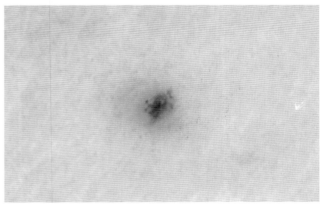

FIGURE 4.113 Combined nevus (dermoscopy)

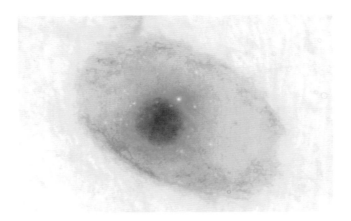

FIGURE 4.114 Combined nevus (dermoscopy)

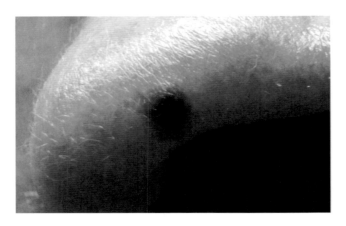

FIGURE 4.115 (a) Deep penetrating nevus (clinical)

Deep penetrating nevi are considered variants of intradermal nevi or blue nevi.

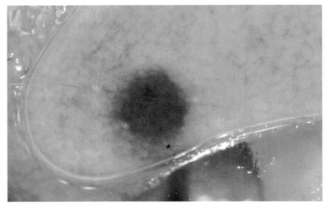

FIGURE 4.115 (b) Deep penetrating nevus (dermoscopy)

Under dermoscopy examination they are either indistinguishable from blue nevi (uniform blue pigmentation) or, as in this case, may have additional colors.

CHAPTER FIVE

MELANOMA

Lentigo maligna (Hutchinson's melanotic freckle)

Lentigo maligna (Hutchinson's melanotic freckle) is an in situ melanoma occurring on chronically sun-exposed sites, usually the head and neck. Classically, they are seen as enlarging and irregularly pigmented macules. Histopathologically, neoplastic melanocytes are seen confined within the epidermis. An atrophic epidermis commonly occurs on a background of dermal solar elastosis. Melanophages are common.

Because of its great morphological variability, lentigo maligna is perhaps the most difficult diagnostic group in dermoscopy. Varying degrees of in situ melanoma can occur, ranging from single melanoma cells to intraepidermal nests. Thus, lentigo maligna can range from being light (tan) in color to being heavily pigmented. In addition, varying degrees of epidermal atrophy can lead to a spectrum from no pigmented network (uncommon) to a prominent, irregularly broadened network forming rhomboidal structures (classic form). However, due to the presence of dilated hair follicles on the face, many benign pigmented macules can also have a pseudo broadened network. The network of a benign lesion is usually not prominent.

The dermoscopic features of lentigo maligna[1] are:

- irregular prominent (dark) broadened network (common)
- rhomboidal structures (common)
- asymmetric pigmented follicular openings (common)
- multiple blue-gray dots (common)
- annular granular pattern (common)
- slate gray globules (common)
- dark homogeneous areas (some)
- follicular plugs (some)
- irregular discrete (light) network (some)
- uniform pigment background (some)
- absent blue-white veil, pseudopods, radial streaming

Since pseudopods and radial streaming histopathologically represent the radial growth phase of melanoma, on initial inspection it is surprising to observe that lentigo maligna, which is a lesion purely in the radial growth phase, lacks pseudopods and radial streaming. However, in general, the major histopathological finding of lentigo maligna is the presence of single melanoma cells and small nests of melanoma cells, usually at the basal layer. This is in contrast to the confluent intraepidermal radial nests seen when pseudopods and radial streaming are present in superficial spreading melanoma.[2]

Lentigo maligna melanoma

Some lentigo maligna progress to invasive melanoma (lentigo maligna melanoma). The dermoscopic findings of lentigo maligna melanoma are of invasive melanoma (see below) on a background of lentigo maligna (see above).

Superficial spreading and nodular melanoma ("invasive melanoma")

Superficial spreading melanoma is defined histologically as an invasive melanoma (dermal invasion of neoplastic melanocytes arising from the epidermis) with intraepidermal involvement in the radial growth phase at least three rete ridges beyond the area of dermal invasion. Nodular melanoma is defined as a vertically invasive melanoma that lacks intraepidermal tumor beyond the margins of the invasive dermal tumor. Multiple histological sections are required to make the classification of nodular melanoma and many superficial spreading melanomas have a nodular component. For this reason, and because of the lack of published series comparing the dermoscopic features of nodular with other varieties of melanoma, the authors prefer to classify both nodular and superficial spreading melanomas together under the term of "invasive melanoma". Nevertheless, nodular melanoma usually lack the features of thin melanoma (broadened network) and radial growth (radial streaming, pseudopods), but preferentially have the features of thick melanoma (blue-white veil and increased vascularity). More importantly, nodular melanoma are also preferentially amelanotic/hypomelanotic compared with superficial spreading melanoma.

The presentation of invasive melanoma is variable. They are often rapidly growing, and irregularly outlined and pigmented plaques, papules, and nodules (often in combination). However, they can also be relatively amelanotic because of either regression or the presence of true amelanotic tumor cells. Under the surface microscope, 40 features are found to be significantly different in invasive melanoma compared with random atypical pigmented lesions. The major surface dermoscopy findings of invasive melanoma are outlined in Table 5.1.

TABLE 5.1 The major dermoscopic features of invasive pigmented melanoma[3]

Feature	Specificity (%)	Sensitivity (%)
Asymmetric pigmentation	46	100
A single color not found	12	100
Blue-white veil	97	51
Multiple brown dots	97	30
Pseudopods	97	23
Radial streaming	96	18
Negative pigment network	95	22
Irregular depigmentation	92	46
Scar-like depigmentation	93	36
Peripheral black dots/globules	92	42
Multiple (5 or 6) colors	92	53
Multiple blue-dots	91	45
Broadened network	86	35
Peripheral light-brown structureless areas*	96	63

* Data was derived from both in situ and thin invasive melanoma[5]

Method for diagnosis of invasive and in situ melanoma (except lentigo maligna)[4]

There have been a number of dermoscopy methods developed for diagnosing melanoma.[6–9] A robust method for diagnosing invasive melanomas is presented here (Menzies method).[4] This method has been repeatedly shown to have an increased sensitivity for the diagnosis of melanoma (incorporating both invasive and in situ lesions) compared with other published methods both in expert and non-expert settings.[7,10–13] In contrast to other methods[14] it also improves the sensitivity for the diagnosis of small diameter melanoma.[15] Using this method, for a melanoma to be diagnosed, it must have *neither*

of the two morphological negative features *and* one or more of the nine positive features (Table 5.2).

The colors scored are tan, dark brown, black, gray, blue, and red. White is not scored. This method has a sensitivity of 92% for melanoma.[4] Therefore 8% of melanomas are dermoscopically featureless. This may be the case with amelanotic/hypomelanotic melanomas or some early invasive pigmented melanomas.

TABLE 5.2 Method for diagnosis of pigmented melanoma (Menzies method)

Negative Features—*CANNOT BE FOUND*

Symmetrical pigmentation pattern

Presence of only a single color

Positive Features—*AT LEAST ONE FEATURE FOUND*

Blue-white veil

Multiple brown dots

Pseudopods

Radial streaming

Scar-like depigmentation

Peripheral black dots/globules

Multiple (5–6) colors

Multiple blue-gray dots

Broadened network

It should be emphasized that, in general, invasive melanomas have disordered architecture (disordered pigmentation pattern) usually to a greater degree than dysplastic nevi or other benign lesions. Finally, since the dermoscopic features of in situ melanoma (non-lentigo maligna) are similar to early invasive melanoma[16], the method in Table 5.2 is accurate for in situ melanoma.

Amelanotic and hypomelanotic melanoma

Pure amelanotic primary melanoma of the skin is rare, with the largest series suggesting an incidence less than 2% of melanomas.[17] However, partially pigmented or light colored (hypomelanotic) melanoma are not as rare. *Amelanotic* lesions have no melanin pigmentation (tan, dark brown, blue, gray, or black) upon dermoscopy inspection. *Partially pigmented* lesions have a surface area of melanin pigmentation upon dermoscopy inspection less than 25% of its total surface. *Light-colored* lesions have only tan, light blue, or light gray pigmentation which may occupy greater than 25% of its total surface area. No dark brown, deep blue, or black color is found. It is important to realize that the conventional 2 step procedure for diagnosing pigmented skin lesions using dermoscopy (see Chapter 7) is relatively ineffective for amelanotic/hypomelanotic melanoma.[18] The major dermoscopic features of amelanotic/hypomelanotic melanoma are outlined in Table 5.3.

TABLE 5.3 The major dermoscopic features of amelanotic/ hypomelanotic melanoma[18]

Feature	Specificity %	Sensitivity %
Negative features		
Multiple (>3) milia-like cysts		1
Comma vessels regular distribution		1
Comma vessels the predominant vessel type		3
Symmetrical pigmentation pattern		8
Irregular size or distributed or multiple blue-gray globules		2–4
Positive features		
Blue-white veil	99	11
Scar-like depigmentation	94	23
Multiple blue-gray dots	93	22
Irregular depigmentation	86	35
Brown dots/globules irregular	91	24
5–6 colors	95	15
Predominant central vessels	94	16
Red-blue color	88	28
Peripheral light-brown structureless areas	93	19

Of the vascular-related features the most predictive for melanoma are in order[18]:

- predominantly central vessels
- hairpin vessels
- milky red pink areas
- greater than one shade of pink
- combination of dotted and linear irregular vessels
- linear irregular vessels as the predominant vessel type

It has been shown to be relatively easier to distinguish all malignant amelanotic/hypomelanotic lesions from all benign lesions (rather than to attempt to discriminate melanoma from other malignant lesions such as BCC). In this regard additional important features are[18]:

- large diameter vessels
- arborising vessels
- ulceration
- gray color

- any pigmented feature of BCC (see Chapter 6)

Finally it is important to realize that while dermoscopy aids in the diagnosis of amelanotic/hypomelanotic melanoma, the diagnostic accuracy is less than that seen with more pigmented melanoma.[18]

Cutaneous metastatic melanoma

Intradermal metastatic melanoma is usually found as local or in-transit metastases (proximal to the primary melanoma site and distal to the regional lymph nodes). Usually they present as firm blue nodules. Because of the lack of epidermal pathology they appear relatively featureless under dermoscopy. Most commonly a homogeneous pigmentation pattern sometimes resembling a blue nevus is found, although amelanotic and saccular patterns are also commonly seen.[19]

When pigmented, colors range from brown-gray (most common), to blue and black. Increased vascularity is seen with "winding" and polymorphous vessels predominating. Finally a pigment halo and peripheral gray spots may also be found.

Acral lentiginous melanoma

Melanoma on the palms and soles, like benign nevi, have a different dermoscopy appearance than on non–volar sites.[20,21] In particular, the macular/flat (often in situ) component of acral lentiginous melanoma usually has distinct pigment network known as the parallel ridge pattern. This occurs in 86% of acral lentiginous melanomas with a very high specificity of 99%.[20] Irregular diffuse pigmentation with variable shades from tan to black is also an important diagnostic feature with an 85% sensitivity and 97% specificity for the diagnosis of acral melanoma.[20]

The dermoscopy features of the invasive melanoma components of acral lentiginous melanoma become more like classical non-volar melanoma (Table 5.2) as the Breslow depth increases. It should also be noted that a proportion of volar melanoma are amelanotic. The dermoscopic features of acral lentiginous melanoma[20,21,22] are:

- asymmetric pigmentation pattern (common)
- parallel ridge pattern (macular/in situ component) (common)
- irregular diffuse pigmentation (common)
- irregularly distributed brown or black globules (some)
- classical features of invasive melanoma (raised component) (common)

- lack of parallel furrow, lattice, or regular fibrillar/filamentous patterns uniformly throughout the lesion (universal)

Saida et al. has additionally proposed that all lesions with a diameter greater than 7 mm without the typical parallel furrow, lattice or uniform fibrillar patterns be biopsied.[23]

Subungual melanoma and its differential diagnosis

Subungual melanoma (melanoma arising from the nail matrix) occurs in a frequent proportion of melanomas in the African, Native American, and Asian races (20%).[24] In contrast they occur in a much lower proportion of melanomas in light-skinned races (1%). In the early stages they present as a pigmented stripe of the nail plate (longitudinal melanonychia) with an enlarging width. The dermoscopic features of subungual melanoma are[25]:

- brown background (very common)
- irregular brown to black lines (very common)
- micro-Hutchinson's sign (some)
- nail dystrophy or destruction (when invasive)
- blood spots (later sign)

The brown bands within longitudinal melanonychia establishing a diagnosis of a proliferative melanocytic lesion of the nail matrix (nevus or melanoma) are significantly more irregular in width, color, spacing, and parallelism in melanoma. However, a history of an overall increasing width of longitudinal melanonychia is also a key to the early diagnosis of subungual melanoma. Extension of pigmentation on or beyond the proximal or lateral nail folds (Hutchinson's sign) is a later sign. Nail dystrophy or destruction usually indicates the onset of invasion.

Finally, the position of the pigment at the free edge of the nail plate under dermoscopic examination can help determine the location of the lesion within the nail matrix and aid the diagnostic biopsy.[26] Pigment in the lower half of the nail plate indicates that the lesion lies in the distal matrix, and pigment in the upper half of the nail plate indicates the lesion lies in the proximal matrix. Such an observation allows accurate matrix biopsy sometimes reducing nail dystrophy (since biopsy of the distal matrix will induce less nail damage).

Subungual nevi also present as longitudinal melanonychia. The dermoscopic features of subungual nevi are[25]:

- brown background (very common)
- regular brown lines (very common)

Subungual melanotic macules (most commonly due to a lentigo, ethnic (dark-skinned races), medications, endocrine disorders, or repetitive trauma) present as longitudinal melanoncyhia due to increased melanin production without proliferation of nail matrix melanocytes. These all have the same dermoscopic features of[25,27]:

- gray background (very common)
- regular gray lines (very common)
- brown background (few)

Subungual lentigo are normally solitary in contrast to the multiple nature of ethnic, endocrine, and drug-induced nail lesions.

Subungual hemorrhages are usually very easily distinguished from the above diagnoses due to the dermoscopic features of:

- blood spots (near universal)
- red-blue homogeneous areas (common)
- absence of longitudinal brown, gray or black lines extending the full length of the nail (universal)
- increasing sparing (no pigmentation) of the proximal nail over time (universal)

The color of blood spots and the more extensive homogeneous areas are most commonly red to red-blue or black but sometimes may be brown. Rarely, when a subungual hemorrhage does not grow out of the nail or recurs in the same position, a bony exostosis may be the precipitating factor. This can be confirmed by radiological examination of the distal phalynx. If the diagnosis cannot be established biopsy is indicated.[27] Finally, nail pigmentation can be caused by fungal or bacterial infections, with microbiological culture confirming the diagnosis.

References

1. Schiffner, R, Schiffner-Rohe, J, Vogt, T, Landthaler, M, Wlotzke, U, Cognetta, A, Stolz, W. Improvement of early recognition of lentigo maligna using dermatoscopy. *J Am Acad Dermatol* 2000; 42: 25–32.

2. Menzies, S, Crotty, K, McCarthy, W. The morphologic criteria of the pseudopod in surface microscopy. *Arch Dermatol* 1995; 131: 436–40.

3. Menzies, S, Ingvar, C, McCarthy, W. A sensitivity and specificity analysis of the surface microscopy features of invasive melanoma. *Melanoma Res* 1996; 6: 55–62.

4. Menzies, S, Ingvar, C, Crotty, K, McCarthy, W. Frequency and morphologic characteristics of invasive melanomas lacking specific surface microscopic features. *Arch Dermatol* 1996; 132: 1178–82.

INDEX

Page numbers in *italics* refer to illustrations.

5. Annessi, G. Bono, R. Sampogna, F. Faraggiana, T. Abeni, D. Sensitivity, specificity, and diagnostic accuracy of three dermoscopic algorithmic methods in the diagnosis of doubtful melanocytic lesions: the importance of light brown structureless areas in differentiating atypical melanocytic nevi from thin melanomas. *J Am Acad Dermatol* 2007; 56:759–67.

6. Soyer, H. Argenziano, G. Chimenti, S. Menzies, S. Pehamberger, H. Rabinovitz, H. Stolz, W. Kopf, A. *Dermoscopy of Pigmented Skin Lesions*. Milan, Italy: Edra: 2001.

7. Blum, A. Rassner, G. Garbe, C. Modified ABC-point list of dermoscopy: A simplified and highly accurate dermoscopic algorithm for the diagnosis of cutaneous melanocytic lesions. *J Am Acad Dermatol* 2003; 48:672–8.

8. Zalaudek, I. Argenziano, G. Soyer, HP. et al. Three-point checklist of dermoscopy: an open internet study. *Br J Dermatol* 2006; 154:431–7.

9. Henning, JS. Dusza, SW. Wang, SQ. et al. The CASH (color, architecture, symmetry, and homogeneity) algorithm for dermoscopy. *J Am Acad Dermatol* 2007; 56:45–52.

10. Argenziano, G. Soyer, HP. Chimenti, S. et al. Dermoscopy of pigmented skin lesions: results of a consensus meeting via the internet. *J Am Acad Dermatol* 2003; 48:679–93.

11. Dolianitis, C. Kelly, J. Wolfe, R. Simpson, P. Comparative performance of 4 dermoscopic algorithms by nonexperts for the diagnosis of melanocytic lesions. *Arch Dermatol* 2005; 141:1008–14.

12. Blum, A. Leudtke, H. Ellwanger, U. Schwabe, R. Rassner, G. Garbe, C. Digital image analysis for diagnosis of cutaneous melanoma. Development of a highly effective computer algorithm based on analysis of 837 melanocytic lesions. *Br J Dermatol* 2004; 151: 1029–38.

13. Henning, JS. Stein, J. Yeung, J. et al. CASH algorithm for dermoscopy revisited. *Arch Dermatol* 2008; 144: 554–5.

14. Carli, P. De Giorgi, V. Chiarugi, A. et al. Effect of lesion size on the diagnostic performance of dermoscopy in melanoma detection. *Dermatology* 2003; 206:292–6.

15. Bono, A. Tolomio, E. Trincone, S. et al. Micro-melanoma detection: a clinical study on 206 consecutive cases of pigmented skin lesions with a diameter < or = 3 mm. *Br J Dermatol* 2006; 155: 570–3.

16. Pizzichetta, MA. Argenziano, G. Talamini, R. et al. Dermoscopic criteria for melanoma in situ are similar to those for early invasive melanoma. *Cancer* 2001 (Mar 1); 91(5): 992–7.

17. Giuliano, AE. Cochran, A. Morton, D. Melanoma from unknown primary site and amelanotic melanoma. *Seminars Oncol* 1982; 9: 442–7.

18. Menzies, SW. Kreusch, J. Byth, K. Pizzichetta, MD. et al. Dermoscopy of amelanotic and hypomelanotic melanoma. *Arch Dermatol* 2008; 114: 1120–7.

19. Bono, R. Giampetruzzi, AR. Concolino, F. Puddu, P. Scoppola, A. Sera, F. Marchetti, P. Dermoscopic patterns of cutaneous melanoma metastases. *Melanoma Res* 2004; 14: 367–73.

20. Saida, T. Miyazaki, A. Oguchi, S. Ishihara, Y. et al. Significance of dermoscopic patterns in detecting malignant melanoma on acral volar skin: results of a multicenter study in Japan. *Arch Dermatol* 2004; 140: 1233–8.

21. Saida, T. Oguchi, S. Ishihara, Y. In vivo observation of magnified features of pigmented lesions on volar skin using video macroscope. *Arch Dermatol* 1995; 131: 298–304.

22. Altamura, D. Altobelli, E. Micantonio, T. Piccolo, D. Fargnoli, MC. Peris, K. Dermoscopic patterns of acral melanocytic nevi and melanomas in a white population in central Italy. *Arch Dermatol* 2006; 142: 1123–8.

23. Saida, T. Koga, H. Dermoscopic patterns of acral melanocytic nevi: their variations, changes, and significance. *Arch Dermatol* 2007; 143: 1423–6.

24. Levit, E. Kagen, M. Scher, R. Grossman, M. Altman, E. The ABC rule for clinical detection of subungual melanoma. *J Am Acad Dermatol* 2000; 42: 269–74.

25. Ronger, S. Touzet, S. Ligeron, C. Balme, B. Viallard, AM. Barrut, D. Colin, C. Thomas, L. Dermoscopic examination of nail pigmentation. *Arch Dermatol* 2002 138: 1327–33.

26. Braun, RP. Baran, R. Saurat, JH. Thomas, L. Surgical Pearl: Dermoscopy of the free edge of the nail to determine the level of nail plate pigmentation and the location of its probable origin in the proximal or distal nail matrix. *J Am Acad Dermatol* 2006; 55: 512–3.

27. Braun, RP. Baran, R. Le Gal, FA. et al. Diagnosis and management of nail pigmentations. *J Am Acad Dermatol* 2007; 56: 835–47.

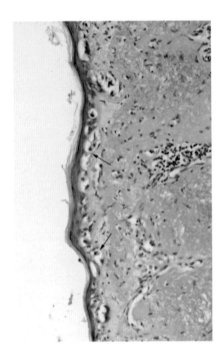

FIGURE 5.1 Lentigo maligna (Hutchinson's melanotic freckle) (histopathology)

This variant of in situ malignant melanoma (melanoma confined to the epidermis) shows confluent large atypical melanocytes with retracted cytoplasm present in the basal layer of the epidermis (arrows). The epidermis is atrophic and the dermis shows evidence of solar damage (solar elastosis). Magnification ×50 (H & E stain).

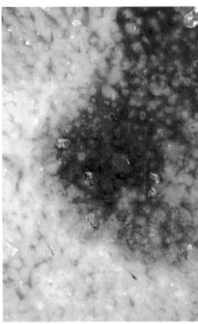

FIGURE 5.2 (b) Lentigo maligna (Hutchinson's melanotic freckle) (dermoscopy)

Under dermoscopy they classically appear with areas of irregular, broadened network, which may be heavily pigmented forming rhomboidal structures (a more specific finding, seen centrally in the figure) or tan in color. Note the multiple follicular plugs and slate gray globules (bottom right) which are also features of lentigo maligna.

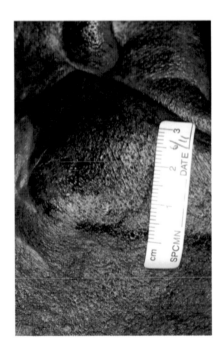

FIGURE 5.2 (a) Lentigo maligna (Hutchinson's melanotic freckle) (clinical view)

Lentigo maligna classically appear as radial growing, irregularly dark pigmented macules of heavily sun-exposed sites, usually the head and neck.

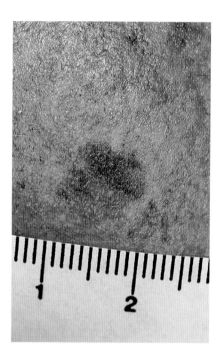

FIGURE 5.3 (a) Lentigo maligna (Hutchinson's melanotic freckle) (clinical view)

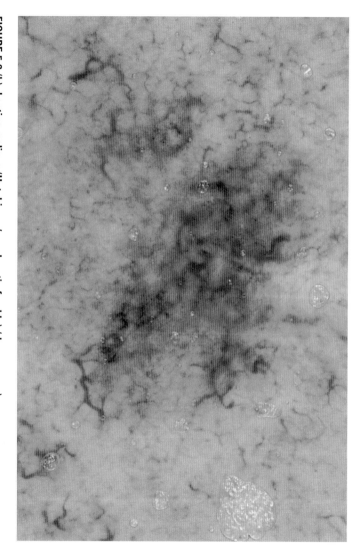

FIGURE 5.3 (b) Lentigo maligna (Hutchinson's melanotic freckle) (dermoscopy)

Here multiple blue-gray dots form a pseudo-broadened network with the holes of the network formed by follicular openings. Melanophages are common in lentigo maligna. Interfollicular multiple blue-gray dots (melanophages) or dark brown dots (due to intraepidermal melanoma cells) may form annular granular structures as seen scattered throughout this lesion.

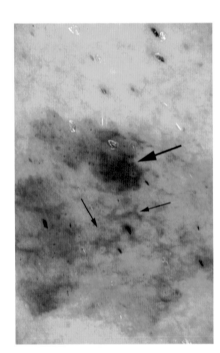

FIGURE 5.4 Lentigo maligna (Hutchinson's melanotic freckle) (dermoscopy)

Areas of prominent gray broadened network (small arrows) and dark homogenous areas (large arrow) characterize this lesion as lentigo maligna. As the density of melanoma cells increases in the epidermis the broadened network forming rhomboidal structures are replaced by more homogeneous pigmentation.

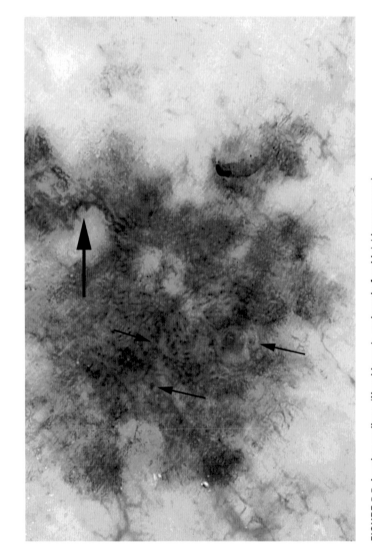

FIGURE 5.5 Lentigo maligna (Hutchinson's melanotic freckle) (dermoscopy)

Here slate gray globules are seen (small arrows) on a background of an irregular network with focal broadening (large arrow). Slate gray globules form from accumulations of melanophages high in the dermis.

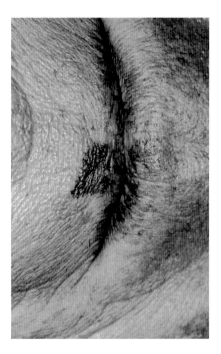

FIGURE 5.6 (a) Lentigo maligna (Hutchinson's melanotic freckle) (clinical view)

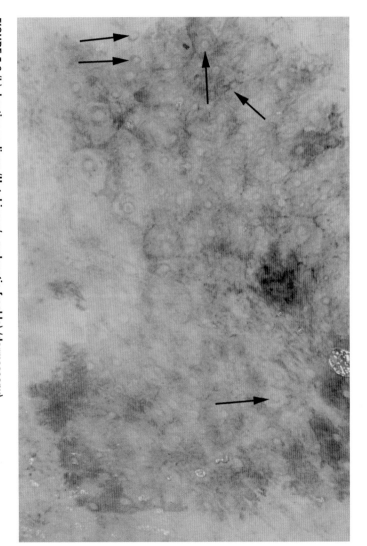

FIGURE 5.6 (b) Lentigo maligna (Hutchinson's melanotic freckle) (dermoscopy)
Areas of asymmetric pigmented follicular openings are seen in this lesion (arrows).

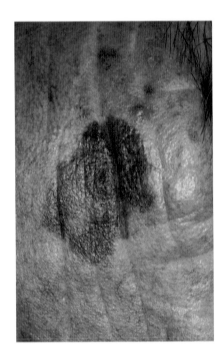

FIGURE 5.7 (a) Lentigo maligna (Hutchinson's melanotic freckle) (clinical view)

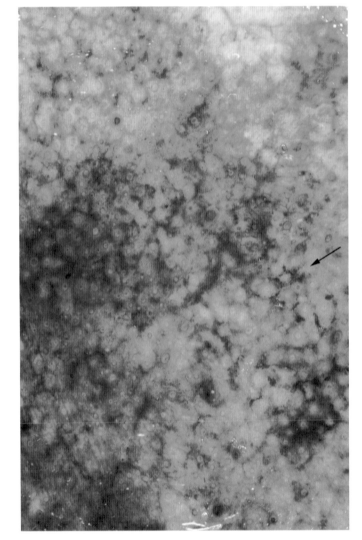

FIGURE 5.7 (b) Lentigo maligna (Hutchinson's melanotic freckle) (dermoscopy)
Areas of irregular, prominent, broadened network, forming rhomboidal structures (bottom left) define this lentigo maligna. There are also slate gray globules and occasional asymmetric pigmented follicular openings within the lesion. Also note the annular granular structures formed by interfollicular multiple blue-gray dots (arrow).

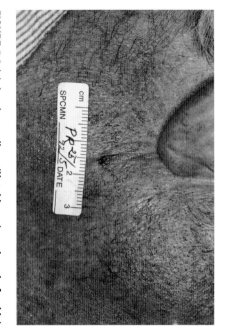

FIGURE 5.8 (a) **Lentigo maligna (Hutchinson's melanotic freckle) (clinical view)**

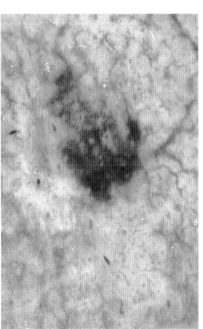

FIGURE 5.8 (b) **Lentigo maligna (Hutchinson's melanotic freckle) (dermoscopy)**

Here a pseudo-broadened network is formed from multiple blue dots (melanophages).

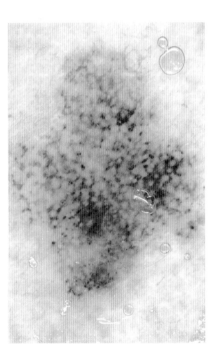

FIGURE 5.9 **Lentigo maligna (Hutchinson's melanotic freckle) (dermoscopy)**

While lentigo maligna is a purely epidermal (in situ) melanoma, pseudopods and radial streaming (intraepidermal confluent radial nests of melanoma) are rarely seen. This is because the epidermal involvement of tumor in lentigo maligna tends to be single cell (or small groups of cells) compared with the confluent radial nests seen in many superficial spreading melanomas.

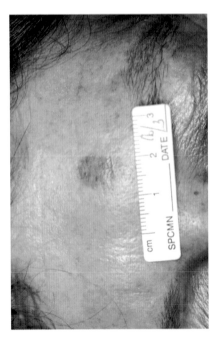

FIGURE 5.10 (a) Lentigo maligna (Hutchinson's melanotic freckle) (clinical view)

Lentigo maligna can be very variable in its clinical appearance. Here it presents as a growing tan macule.

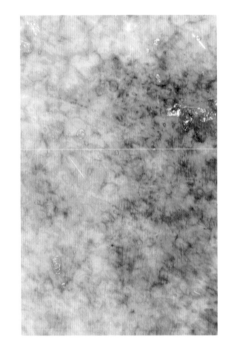

FIGURE 5.10 (b) Lentigo maligna (Hutchinson's melanotic freckle) (dermoscopy)

The dermoscopic features of lentigo maligna are also extremely variable. No evidence of a broadened network is seen within this discrete (lightly pigmented) network. Indeed, much of this lesion contains only a uniformly pigmented background. This lesion was subjected to biopsy because it was enlarging.

FIGURE 5.11 Lentigo maligna (Hutchinson's melanotic freckle) (dermoscopy)

Again, no broadened network is seen here. Because of the great morphological variability seen in lentigo maligna, it is perhaps the most difficult diagnostic group in dermoscopy. Varying degrees of in situ melanoma can occur, from a few melanoma cells at the base of the epidermis to intraepidermal nests. Therefore, lentigo maligna can range in color from tan to heavily pigmented.

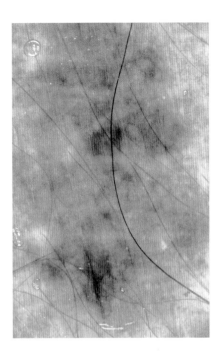

FIGURE 5.12 Lentigo maligna (Hutchinson's melanotic freckle) (dermoscopy)

This lesion has scattered asymmetric pigmented follicular openings and areas of more prominent network.

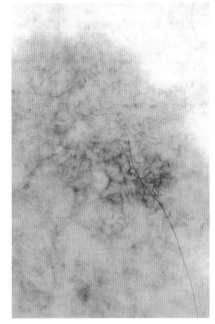

FIGURE 5.13 Lentigo maligna (Hutchinson's melanotic freckle) (dermoscopy)

In lentigo maligna, varying degrees of epidermal atrophy can lead to a spectrum from no pigment network (less common) to a prominent, irregularly broadened network (classic form). In this presentation of lentigo maligna no pigment network can be seen.

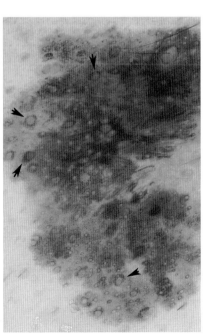

FIGURE 5.14 Lentigo maligna (dermoscopy)

Here many asymmetric pigmented follicular openings are seen throughout the lesion (arrows).

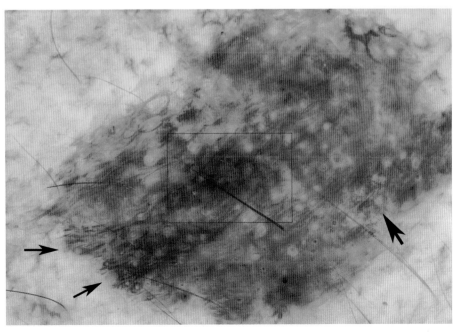

FIGURE 5.15 Lentigo maligna (dermoscopy)

While some fingerprint-like areas are seen in part of the lesion (thin arrows) loosely formed rhomboid structures (within the rectangle) favor the diagnosis of lentigo maligna. Note also the areas of multiple blue-gray dots (large arrow).

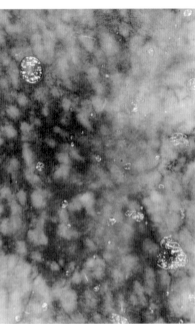

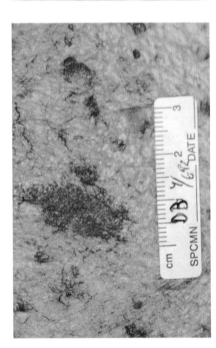

FIGURE 5.16 (a) Lentigo maligna melanoma (clinical view)
Lentigo maligna may progress to invasive melanoma (lentigo maligna melanoma). In their early stages of invasion lentigo maligna melanoma appear identical to their in situ counterpart.

FIGURE 5.16 (b) Lentigo maligna melanoma (dermoscopy)
Areas of gray/blue broadened network suggest the possibility of dermal invasion. However, in many cases, this may be due to pigment incontinence (melanophages) (0.4 mm Breslow depth).

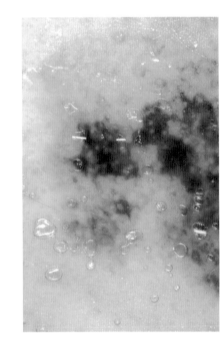

FIGURE 5.17 Lentigo maligna melanoma (dermoscopy)
Small confluent areas of blue pigmentation suggest the possibility of progression to invasive melanoma (0.4 mm Breslow depth).

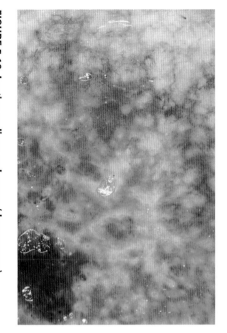

FIGURE 5.18 Lentigo maligna melanoma (dermoscopy)
Scar-like depigmentation indicates the possibility of invasion (1.0 mm Breslow depth).

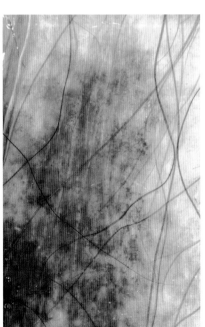

FIGURE 5.19 Lentigo maligna melanoma (dermoscopy)
Multiple blue dots (melanophages) indicate gross regression of this lentigo maligna melanoma (0.3 mm Breslow depth).

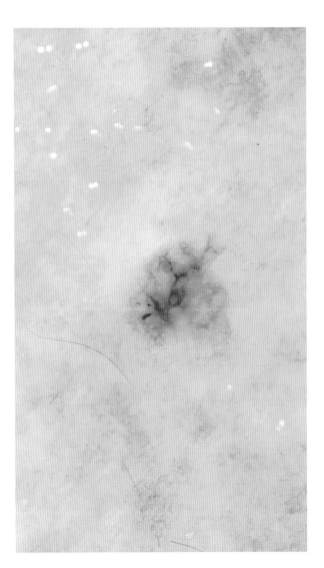

FIGURE 5.20 In situ melanoma (dermoscopy)
A method is described in Table 5.2 for the diagnosis of pigmented melanoma (non-lentigo maligna). Here this small diameter lesion has neither of the two negative features (symmetry of pigmentation pattern and a single color) and has one positive feature of focal broadened network. This feature is perhaps the most important for the diagnosis of early melanoma.

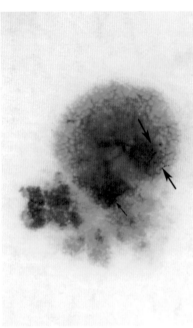

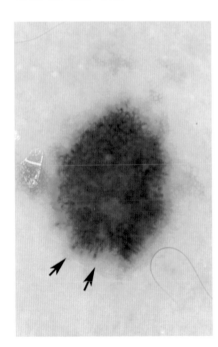

FIGURE 5.21 In situ melanoma (dermoscopy)

This lesion has asymmetry of pattern and more than one color and the positive feature of radial streaming and pseudopods (arrows). The blue structures centrally are globular in structure and hence not satisfying the definition of blue-white veil. Diagnosis: In situ melanoma arising in a compound dysplastic nevus.

FIGURE 5.22 In situ melanoma (dermoscopy)

This multicolored (tan and dark brown) and asymmetric patterned lesion has the positive features of multiple brown dots (delineated by the large arrows) and focal broadened network (small arrow).

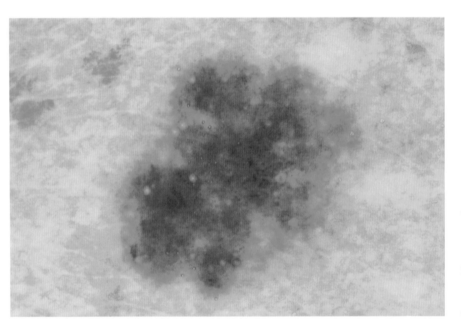

FIGURE 5.23 In situ melanoma (dermoscopy)

This lesion has the positive features of multiple blue-gray dots (granularity). As seen in Chapter 4, small areas of multiple blue-gray dots can occur in nevi. However, this lesion has 50% of its area with blue-gray dots making biopsy essential. Nevertheless, sometimes there can be difficulty in distinguishing such lesions from lichen planus-like keratoses (see Figs 6.62–6.64). Note the white round structures are due to photographic artefact. Diagnosis: Early melanoma in situ arising in a dysplastic junctional nevus.

FIGURE 5.24 In situ melanoma (dermoscopy)

Surprisingly, blue-white veil can occur in some in situ melanoma (as seen centrally here). In these cases it is usually due to a high density of melanophages in combination with increased thickening of the stratum corneum (compact orthokeratosis).

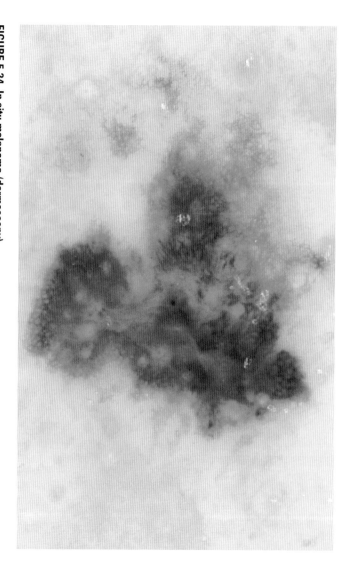

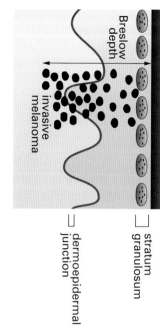

FIGURE 5.25 Breslow depth

Breslow depth is the vertical depth of invasive melanoma, measured from the stratum granulosum of the epidermis to the deepest melanoma cell. Melanomas with a Breslow depth <0.75 mm have a 95% cure rate following excision. Those with a depth >4.0 mm have a mortality of approximately 50%.

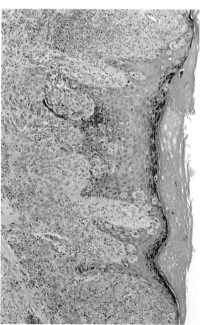

FIGURE 5.26 Invasive melanoma (histopathology)

This invasive melanoma shows neoplastic melanocytes in the epidermis and dermis. The histological diagnosis of malignant melanoma is based on both cytological and architectural features. Melanomas often have an asymmetrical architecture. Most show atypical melanocytes throughout the full thickness of the epidermis. (In nevi there is usually no or minimal atypia and the melanocytes are usually located in the basal layer of the epidermis.) In invasive melanomas there are atypical melanocytes present in the dermis and occasionally in the subcutaneous tissue. These atypical cells are usually larger than nevus cells. Their nuclei are large and have irregular borders. Mitoses are often present in the dermal tumor. There is no single criterion that can be used to diagnose malignant melanoma, and distinguishing histologically between a melanoma and a nevus can be difficult in some cases. It is important that the entire lesion be removed for histological diagnosis, since in many melanocytic lesions areas of malignancy occur focally with surrounding areas appearing benign. Magnification ×25 (H & E stain).

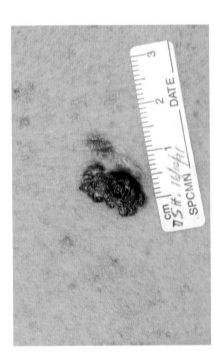

FIGURE 5.27 (a) Invasive melanoma (clinical view)
In its classical form, invasive melanoma is a rapidly growing, darkly pigmented, irregularly shaped lesion.

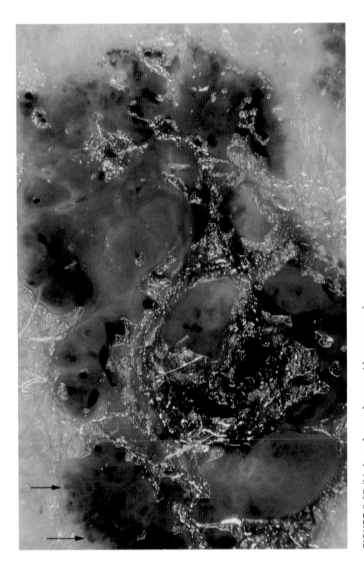

FIGURE 5.27 (b) Invasive melanoma (dermoscopy)
Dermoscopy greatly improves the diagnostic certainty of invasive melanoma. A suggested method for diagnosis which involves observing at least one of nine positive features, in addition to the absence of two negative features, is shown in the introduction to this chapter. This method has a sensitivity of 92% and a specificity of 70% for the diagnosis of invasive melanoma. In this lesion, both of the negative features (single color and symmetrical pigmentation pattern) are absent, and four positive features are found; blue-white veil, pseudopods (arrows), peripheral black dots/globules and multiple (5–6) colors. Colors scored are tan, dark brown, gray, blue, black and red. White is not scored (1.8 mm Breslow depth).

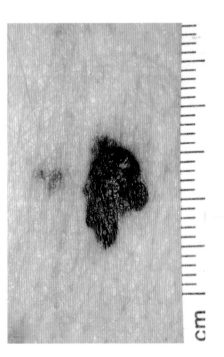

FIGURE 5.28 (a) Invasive melanoma (clinical view)
Many melanomas are clinically multicolored, compared with the limited range of black and brown tones seen in most melanocytic nevi.

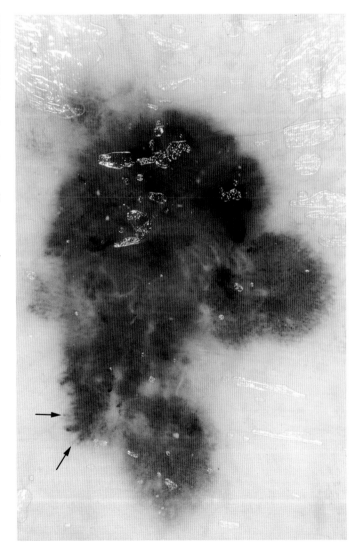

FIGURE 5.28 (b) Invasive melanoma (dermoscopy)
This lesion has absent negative features and the positive features of multiple colors, scar like depigmentation, radial streaming (arrows), blue-white veil, and multiple blue-gray dots (1.3 mm Breslow depth).

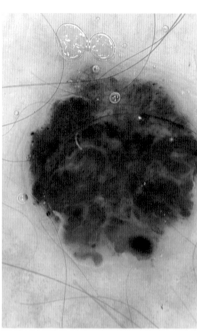

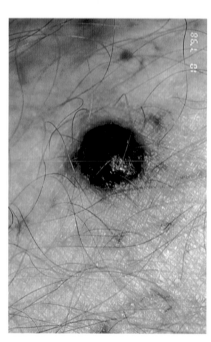

FIGURE 5.29 (a) Invasive melanoma—nodular (clinical view)

FIGURE 5.29 (b) Invasive melanoma—nodular (dermoscopy)

While we have generally incorporated both superficial spreading and nodular melanoma under "invasive" melanoma, pigmented nodular melanomas usually present with absent negative features and at least one positive feature—blue-white veil. In addition, this nodular melanoma has the positive features of multiple colors, scar-like depigmentation and peripheral black dots/globules (2.5 mm Breslow depth).

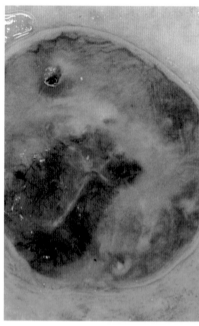

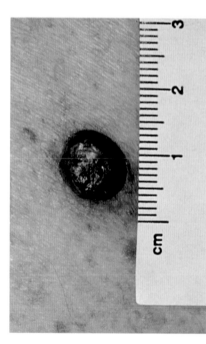

FIGURE 5.30 (a) Invasive melanoma—nodular (clinical view)

FIGURE 5.30 (b) Invasive melanoma—nodular (dermoscopy)

This pigmented nodular melanoma has absent negative features (single color and symmetrical pigmentation pattern) and the distinct positive feature of blue-white veil. Note the increased vascularity seen in many nodular melanomas. The authors have seen only one case of a pigmented nodular melanoma with uniform blue-white veil throughout its entire surface (exhibiting symmetry of pigmentation pattern) (4.0 mm Breslow depth).

FIGURE 5.31 Invasive melanoma—nodular (dermoscopy)
In this rare example of a small diameter nodular melanoma, indistinct areas of blue-white veil centrally led to excision of the lesion (0.9 mm Breslow depth).

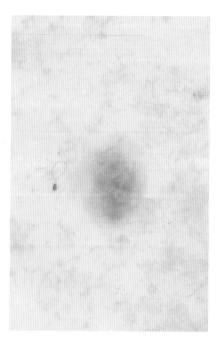

FIGURE 5.32 (a) Invasive melanoma (clinical view)

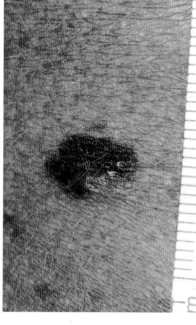

FIGURE 5.32 (b) Invasive melanoma (dermoscopy)
Irregular depigmentation is seen in many invasive melanomas (specificity 92%, sensitivity 46%). It is seen here and includes small areas of the positive feature scar-like depigmentation. Note the relatively regular surrounding pigmentation of the associated dysplastic nevus from which the melanoma has arisen (0.6 mm Breslow depth).

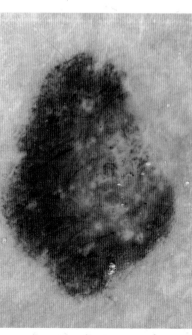

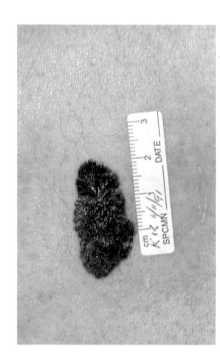

FIGURE 5.33 (a) Invasive melanoma (clinical view)

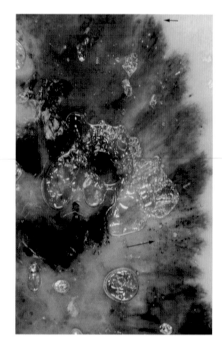

FIGURE 5.33 (b) Invasive melanoma (dermoscopy)
Blue-white veil, multiple brown dots (large arrow) and radial streaming (small arrow) all define this lesion as an invasive melanoma (1.8 mm Breslow depth).

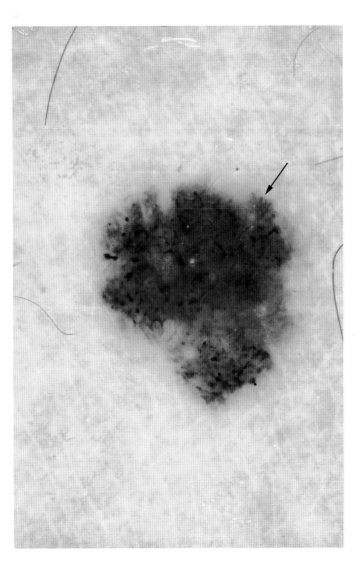

FIGURE 5.34 (b) Invasive melanoma (dermoscopy)
The positive features of pseudopods (arrow) and peripheral black dots/globules (specificity 92%, sensitivity 42%) are seen (0.8 mm Breslow depth).

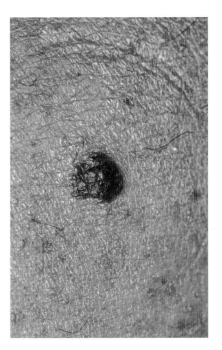

FIGURE 5.34 (a) Invasive melanoma (clinical view)

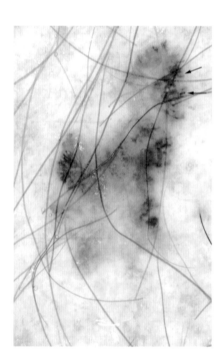

FIGURE 5.35 Invasive melanoma (dermoscopy)
Radial streaming can be a very subtle feature of melanoma. However, here it is quite distinct and plentiful (arrows). Note the extensive regression that obscures most of the dermal component.

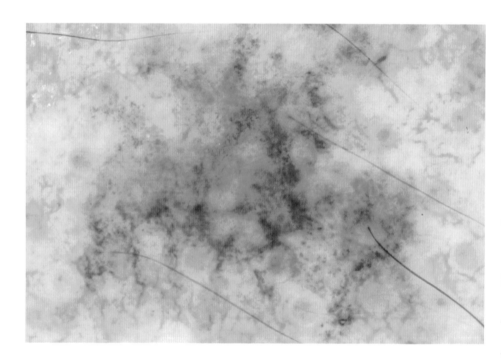

FIGURE 5.36 Invasive melanoma (dermoscopy)
Regression is common in superficial spreading melanoma. The characteristic feature of early regression is the presence of multiple blue-gray dots, which has a specificity of 91% and a sensitivity of 45% for invasive melanoma. In this lesion the solitary finding of areas of uniform tan background and multiple blue-gray dots mimics a lichen planus-like keratosis (see Chapter 6). (0.15 mm Breslow depth).

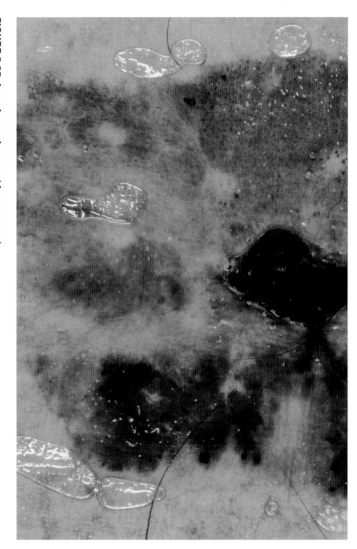

FIGURE 5.37 Invasive melanoma (dermoscopy)
Here multiple colors (specificity 92%, sensitivity 53%), blue-white veil (specificity 97%, sensitivity 51%), peripheral black dots/globules (specificity 92%, sensitivity 42%) and pseudopods (specificity 97%, sensitivity 23%) define this melanoma (1.0 mm Breslow depth).

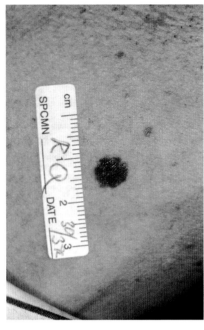

FIGURE 5.38 (a) Invasive melanoma (clinical view)

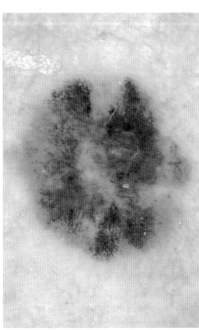

FIGURE 5.38 (b) Invasive melanoma (dermoscopy)
While the pigment network is the unifying feature of melanocyte-derived lesions, using the magnification of the hand-held surface microscope, only 59% of invasive melanomas have a network present. Here, the pigment network confirms its melanocytic origin, while blue-white veil leads to the diagnosis of melanoma (0.4 mm Breslow depth).

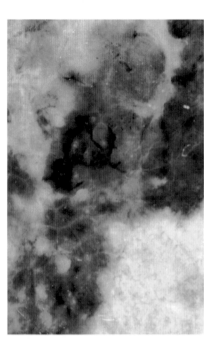

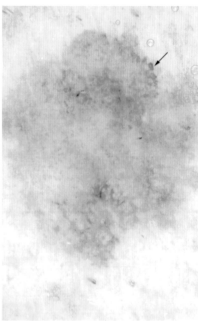

FIGURE 5.41 Invasive melanoma (dermoscopy)
This is a classic example of a multi-colored melanoma (0.7 mm Breslow depth).

FIGURE 5.42 Invasive melanoma (dermoscopy)
This lesion has subtle atypical tan pseudopods (arrow) which lead to the diagnosis of melanoma (0.7 mm Breslow depth).

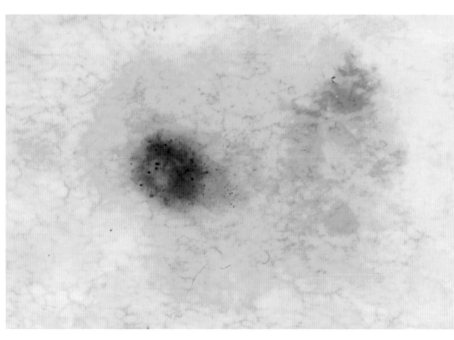

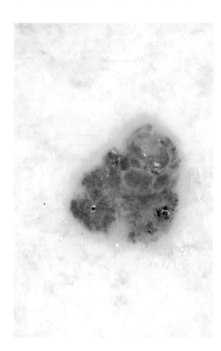

FIGURE 5.39 Invasive melanoma (dermoscopy)
This asymmetric lesion has focal multiple brown dots (0.5 mm Breslow depth).

FIGURE 5.40 Invasive melanoma (dermoscopy)
Not all melanoma are large. This 5 mm diameter lesion has a distinct blue-white veil which leads to the diagnosis of invasive melanoma (1.2 mm Breslow).

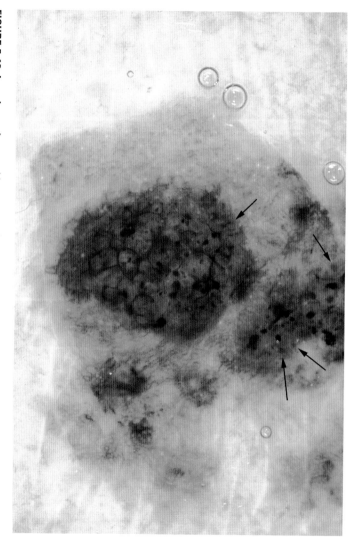

FIGURE 5.43 Invasive melanoma (dermoscopy)

This lesion has pseudopods (arrows) arising at the edge of the melanoma but within the boundary of the nevus from which it has arisen (0.9 mm Breslow depth).

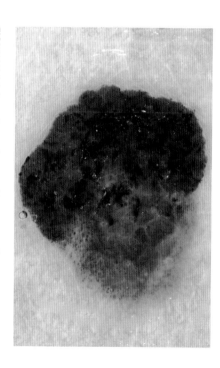

FIGURE 5.44 Invasive melanoma (dermoscopy)

This melanoma has a distinct blue-white veil. Note the associated compound nevus from which it has probably arisen (0.9 mm Breslow depth).

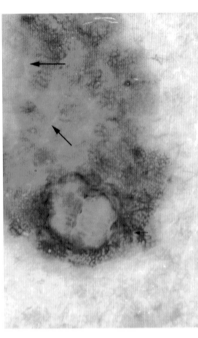

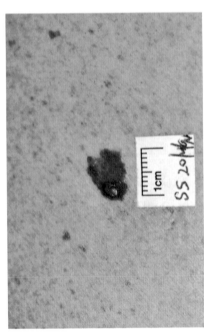

FIGURE 5.45 (a) Invasive melanoma (clinical view)

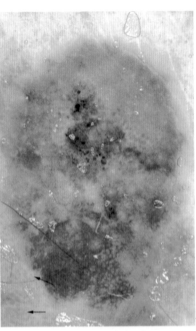

FIGURE 5.45 (b) Invasive melanoma (dermoscopy)
Broadened network in melanoma is usually seen as focally broadened, rather than regularly throughout the lesion. Areas of subtle broadened network (small arrow) (86% specificity, 35% sensitivity) and irregular scar-like depigmentation (large arrows) (93% specificity, 36% sensitivity) can be seen. Note the hypomelanotic nodule of melanoma (0.7 mm Breslow depth).

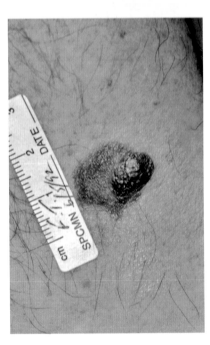

FIGURE 5.46 (a) Invasive melanoma (clinical view)
Here, a nodular melanoma is arising from a superficial spreading melanoma.

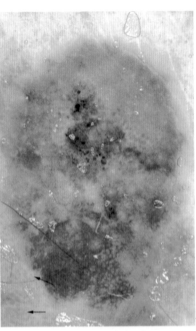

FIGURE 5.46 (b) Invasive melanoma (dermoscopy)
The blue-white veil is so extensive that it almost mimics an area of blue nevus. However, the presence of brown globules and a pigment network makes the diagnosis of melanoma unquestionable. The positive features here are blue-white veil and multiple brown dots (seen as a focal accumulation of dark brown dots near the center of the nodule). Note the areas of negative pigment network (arrows). While this feature is common in Spitz nevi and some dysplastic nevi, it occurs in 22% of melanomas (1.0 mm Breslow depth).

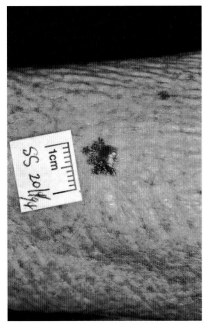

FIGURE 5.48 (a) Invasive melanoma (clinical view)

FIGURE 5.47 Invasive melanoma (dermoscopy)
A large area of negative pigment network can be seen in this melanoma (0.7 mm Breslow depth).

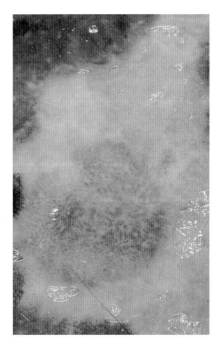

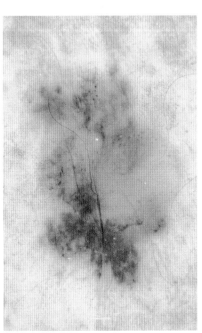

FIGURE 5.48 (b) Invasive melanoma (dermoscopy)
The amelanotic nodule of melanoma is relatively featureless here, and indeed the clinical view is as suggestive that melanoma is the correct diagnosis. Note the subtle pinpoint vessels seen at the periphery of the nodule suggesting its melanocytic origin (1.4 mm Breslow depth).

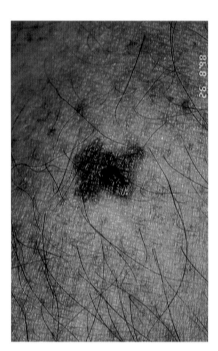

FIGURE 5.49 (a) Invasive melanoma (clinical view)

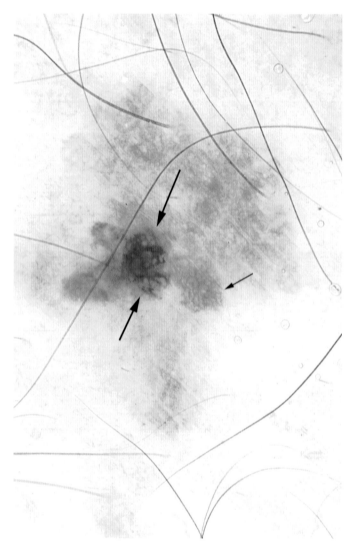

FIGURE 5.49 (b) Invasive melanoma (dermoscopy)

This lesion has absent negative features (single color and symmetrical pigmentation pattern) and one positive feature—broadened network (delineated by large arrows). In melanoma the broadened network is usually only focally found, rather than uniformly distributed throughout the lesion. Note the area of normal network pattern seen elsewhere (small arrow) (0.6 mm Breslow depth).

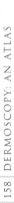

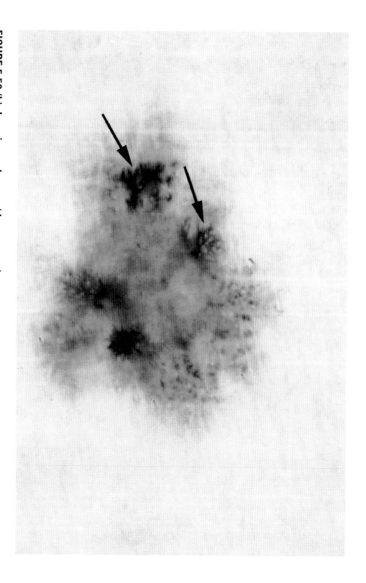

FIGURE 5.50 (b) Invasive melanoma (dermoscopy)

Again a focal broadened network (arrows) characterizes this early invasive melanoma (0.2 mm Breslow depth).

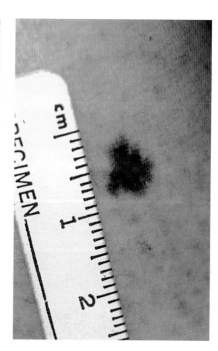

FIGURE 5.50 (a) Invasive melanoma (clinical view)

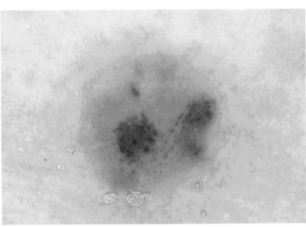

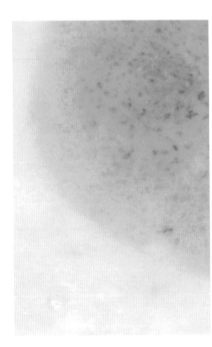

FIGURE 5.51 Amelanotic/hypomelanotic melanoma (dermoscopy)

Pure amelanotic primary melanoma of the skin is rare (less than 2% of melanomas). However, partially pigmented or light colored (hypomelanotic) melanoma are not as uncommon. It is important to realise that the standard two-step procedure for the diagnosis of pigmented skin lesions (see Chapter 7) performs inadequately for amelanotic/hypomelanotic melanoma. The most significant single vascular feature of these melanoma under dermoscopic examination is a predominance of central vessels as seen here (Spindled cell melanoma 0.9 mm Breslow depth).

FIGURE 5.52 Amelanotic/hypomelanotic melanoma (dermoscopy)

Dotted vessels and brown globules confirms the melanocytic origin of the lesion and blue-white veil makes the diagnosis of melanoma. Blue-white veil is the most significant diagnostic feature of amelanotic/hypomelanotic melanoma, however it is only found in 11% of lesions (nodular 2.0 mm Breslow depth).

FIGURE 5.53 Amelanotic/hypomelanotic melanoma (dermoscopy)

Here scar-like depigmentation and large areas of multiple blue-gray dots confirms the diagnosis of melanoma. Note also the peripheral light brown structureless areas occupying more than 10% of the lesion surface. This feature has a specificity of 93% and sensitivity of 19% for the diagnosis of amelanotic/hypomelanotic melanoma (0.55 mm Breslow depth).

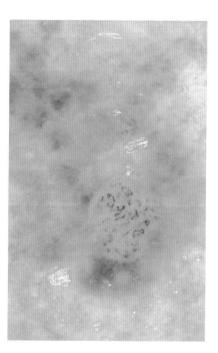

FIGURE 5.54 Amelanotic/hypomelanotic melanoma (dermoscopy)
Here large diameter hairpin vessels characterize the lesion. Amelanotic nodules of melanoma tend to be more vascular than dermal nevi. While hairpin vessels are a significant feature distinguishing melanoma from nevi, they are also found in non-melanocytic lesions. Finally, hairpin vessels are more frequently found in thick versus thin melanoma (1.4 mm Breslow depth).

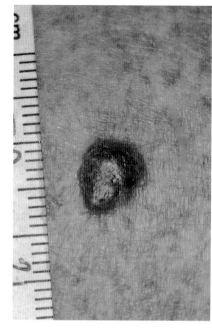

FIGURE 5.55 (a) Amelanotic/hypomelanotic melanoma-nodular (clinical)
A greater proportion of nodular melanoma compared with other subtypes of melanoma are amelanotic/hypomelanotic.

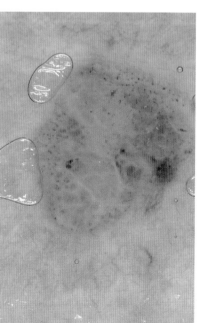

FIGURE 5.55 (b) Amelanotic/hypomelanotic melanoma-nodular (dermoscopy)
Dotted vessels and brown globules confirm this lesion is melanocytic, while blue-white veil and scar-like depigmentation makes the diagnosis of melanoma (2.2 mm Breslow depth).

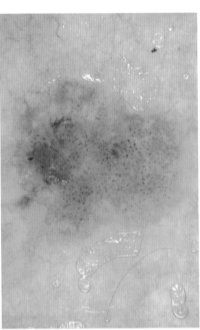

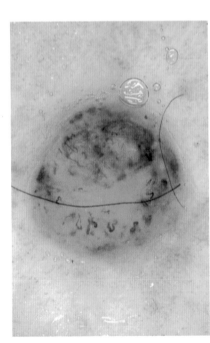

FIGURE 5.56 Amelanotic/hypomelanotic melanoma—nodular (dermoscopy)
Here large diameter vessels that are hairpin in character are seen. In addition, the combination of linear irregular and dotted vessels (top pole of the lesion) are also diagnostic for melanoma (2.2 mm Breslow depth).

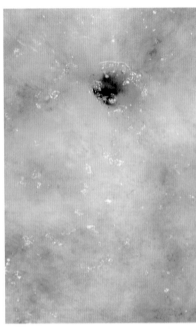

FIGURE 5.57 Amelanotic/hypomelanotic melanoma (dermoscopy)
This lesion has a diffuse tan color that could be ignored with rapid examination. However, dotted vessels confirms the melanocytic origin of the lesion and the presence of predominantly central vessels suggests the need for biopsy (0.9 mm Breslow depth).

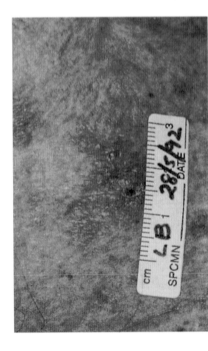

FIGURE 5.58 (a) Amelanotic/hypomelanotic melanoma (clinical)
Amelanotic melanoma can be due to the presence of amelanotic malignant cells or less commonly, as seen here, to extensive regression.

FIGURE 5.58 (b) Amelanotic/hypomelanotic melanoma (dermoscopy)
Under dermoscopic examination areas of widespread irregular scar-like depigmentation and ulceration are seen (0.9 mm Breslow depth).

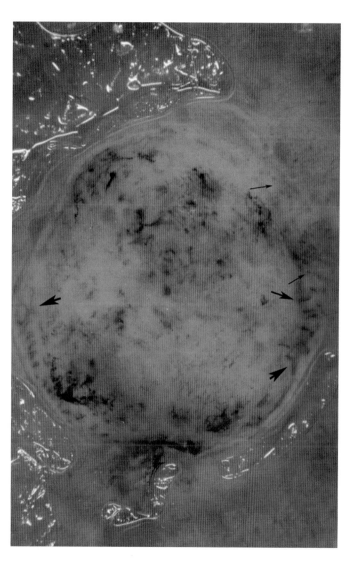

FIGURE 5.59 (b) Amelanotic/hypomelanotic melanoma—nodular (dermoscopy)

In this ulcerated amelanotic nodule, the combination of dotted (small arrow) and linear irregular vessels (thickest arrow) leads to the diagnosis of melanoma. Additionally, hairpin vessels (medium arrow) also favor this diagnosis (2.8 mm Breslow depth).

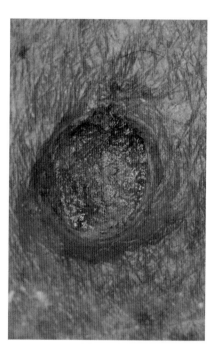

FIGURE 5.59 (a) Amelanotic/hypomelanotic melanoma—nodular (clinical)

FIGURE 5.60 Amelanotic/hypomelanotic melanoma (dermoscopy)
This lesion is characterized by irregular depigmentation, irregularly distributed brown globules, peripheral light-brown structureless areas, milky red-pink areas, and greater than one shade of pink (0.5 mm Breslow thickness with an associated dysplastic junctional nevus).

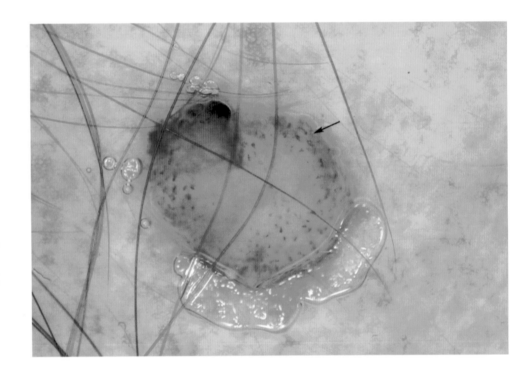

FIGURE 5.61 Amelanotic/hypomelanotic melanoma (dermoscopy)
Here dotted vessels confirm the lesion as melanocytic and the hairpin vessels (arrow) favor melanoma (1.5 mm Breslow thickness).

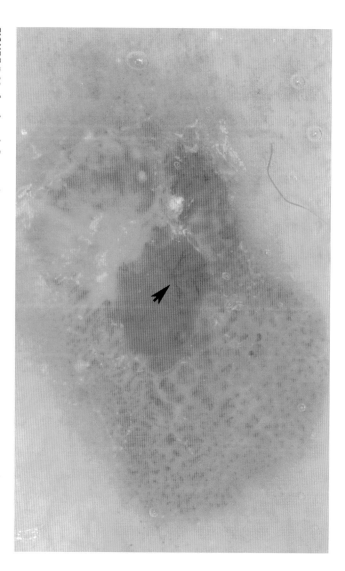

FIGURE 5.63   Amelanotic/hypomelanotic melanoma (dermoscopy)
The dotted vessels confirms the melanocytic origin of the lesion and fine arborizing vessels (arrow); irregular scar-like depigmentation, milky red areas, and more than one shade of pink confirm the diagnosis of melanoma (1.6 mm Breslow depth).

FIGURE 5.62   Amelanotic/hypomelanotic melanoma (dermoscopy)
This lesion has ulceration, a combination of dotted and linear irregular (thick arrow) vessels, hairpin vessels (thin arrow), and more than one shade of pink (2 mm Breslow depth).

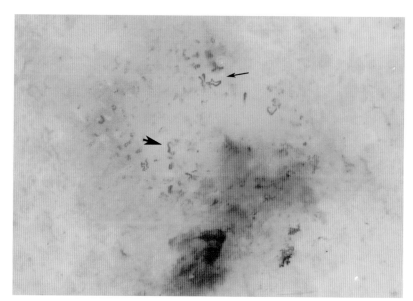

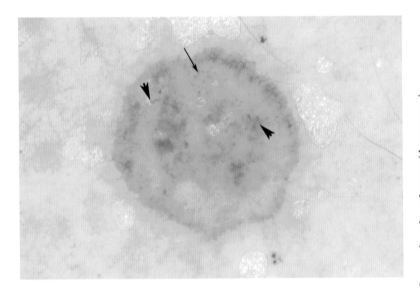

FIGURE 5.64 Amelanotic/hypomelanotic melanoma (dermoscopy)

While this lesion is symmetric in pattern (found in only 8% of amelanotic/hypomelanotic melanoma) it has the significant features of combination of dotted (thin arrow) and linear irregular vessels (thick arrows) (spindled cell 0.7 mm Breslow depth).

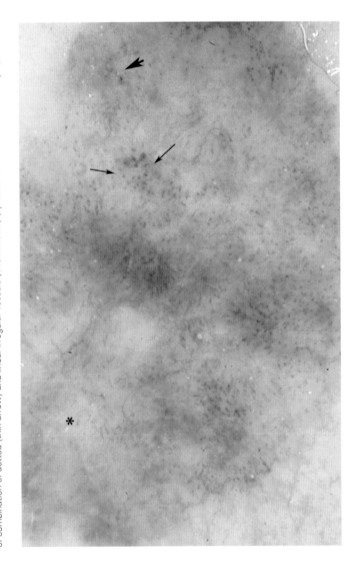

FIGURE 5.65 Amelanotic/hypomelanotic melanoma (dermoscopy)

This lesion has predominant central vessels, greater than one shade of pink, dotted (as delineated by the thin arrows) plus linear irregular vessels (thick arrow) and irregular shaped depigmentation (as indicated by the asterisk). Diagnosis: In situ melanoma arising in a dysplastic nevus.

FIGURE 5.66 Amelanotic/hypomelanotic melanoma (dermoscopy)

This yellow plaque has both fine arborising vessels (thin arrow) and linear irregular vessels (thick arrow). Since there can be an overlap of BCC with amelanotic/hypomelanotic melanoma under dermoscopy examination, the presence of features such as arborizing vessels, ulceration, leaf-like areas, and large blue-gray ovoid nests should always lead to biopsy to confirm the diagnosis (0.8 mm Breslow depth).

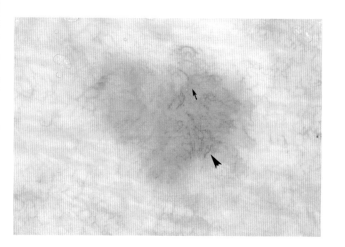

FIGURE 5.67 Amelanotic/hypomelanotic melanoma (dermoscopy)

This light-colored lesion has peripheral light-brown structureless areas, predominant central vessels, and large diameter arborizing vessels. Diagnosis: In situ melanoma.

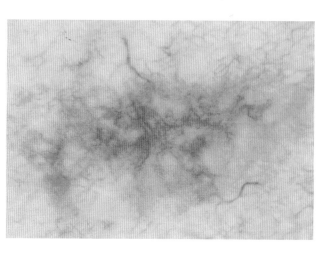

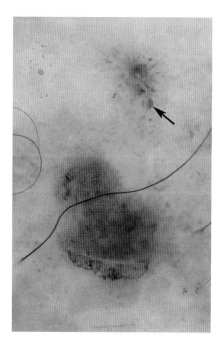

FIGURE 5.68 Amelanotic/hypomelanotic melanoma (dermoscopy)

This lesion has scar-like depigmentation, ulceration, milky red areas, greater than one shade of pink, and milky red globules (arrow). This later feature is only significantly increased in amelanotic/hypomelanotic melanoma compared with non-melanocytic lesions (1.2 mm Breslow depth).

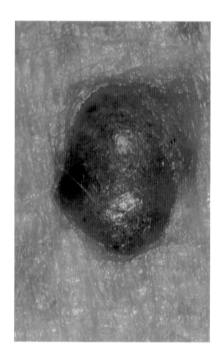

FIGURE 5.69 (a) Amelanotic/hypomelanotic melanoma—nodular (clinical)

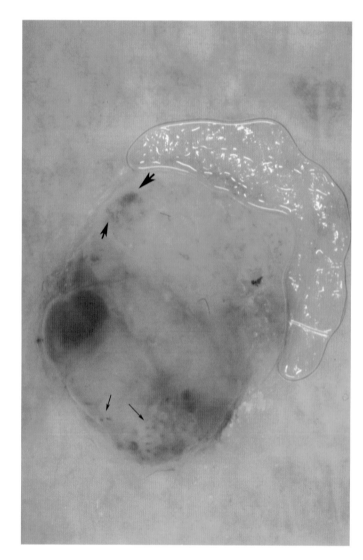

FIGURE 5.69 (b) Amelanotic/hypomelanotic melanoma—nodular (dermoscopy)

While this lesion has an absent network and the presence of large blue-gray ovoid nests indicative of a pigmented BCC, it lacks the vascular features of such a lesion. Specifically the combination of dotted (small arrow) and linear irregular vessels (medium-sized arrow) as well as the milky red globule (large arrow) all lead to the diagnosis of melanoma (nodular melanoma 1.9 mm Breslow depth).

FIGURE 5.70 Amelanotic/hypomelanotic melanoma—nodular (dermoscopy)

This relatively featureless lesion has overlapping features of a dermal nevus (small comma vessels (small arrows) which are the predominant vessel type in only in 3% of amelanotic/hypomelanotic melanoma) and BCC (a large blue-gray ovoid nest; large arrow) (nodular melanoma 2.2 mm Breslow depth).

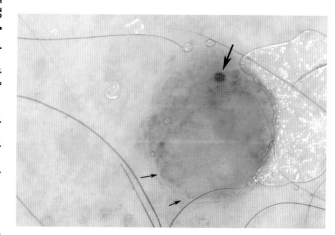

FIGURE 5.71 (a) Invasive melanoma—amelanotic/hypomelanotic (clinical view)

This relatively amelanotic nodule appeared de novo on the lower limb of the patient.

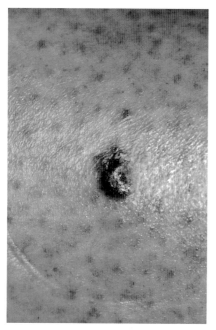

FIGURE 5.71 (b) Invasive melanoma—amelanotic/hypomelanotic (dermoscopy)

Here the lesion has irregularly shaped and distributed brown globules which has a 91% specificity and 24% sensitivity for the diagnosis of amelanotic/hypomelanotic melanoma (0.35 mm Breslow depth).

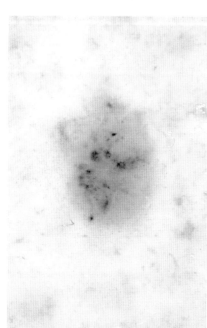

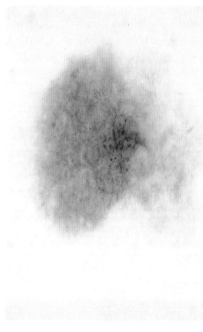

FIGURE 5.72 Invasive melanoma—featureless (dermoscopy)
A small proportion of *pigmented* invasive melanomas have no specific dermoscopic features of melanoma. Fortunately, they tend to be early, thin invasive melanomas, as seen here (0.25 mm Breslow depth).

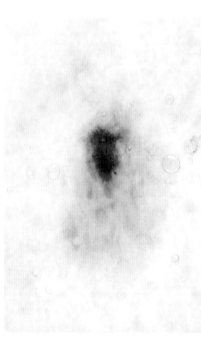

FIGURE 5.73 Invasive melanoma—featureless (dermoscopy)
Note the hair arising in this featureless melanoma. The presence or absence of hair is not a significant finding in invasive melanoma (0.7 mm Breslow depth).

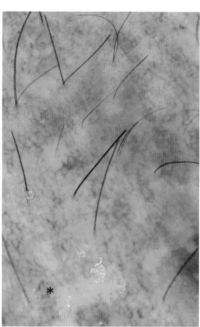

FIGURE 5.74 Invasive melanoma—featureless (dermoscopy)
The discrimination of such featureless melanoma from dysplastic nevi often occurs following changes in digitally monitored nevi (see Chapter 8).

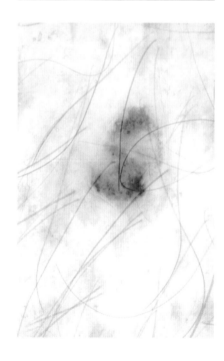

FIGURE 5.75 Invasive melanoma—featureless (dermoscopy)
This tan lesion has a very benign appearance with uniform pigmentation pattern and regular hairs with perifollicular depigmentation. It was excised because of the history of a new lesion on the neck of a male in his late 40s. Nevi of this size are rare to appear as new lesions at this age. Note the non-tumoral vessels which occur on the surrounding skin (asterisk) and throughout the lesion (0.85 mm Breslow depth).

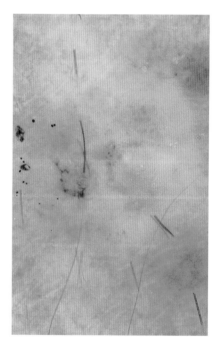

FIGURE 5.76 Invasive melanoma—featureless (dermoscopy)

This dermoscopically featureless pale plaque (albeit with a small area of ulceration) appeared over a few months. Diagnosis: 1.2 mm Desmoplastic melanoma.

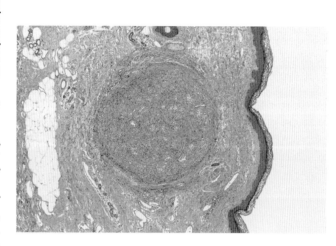

FIGURE 5.77 Invasive melanoma—cutaneous intradermal metastasis (histopathology)

This section shows a nodule of malignant melanoma cells in the dermis. There is no connection with the overlying epidermis. Magnification ×10 (H & E stain).

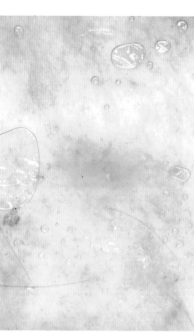

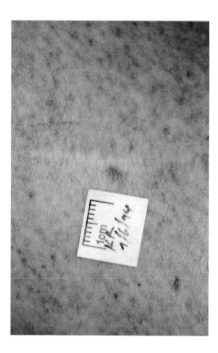

FIGURE 5.78 (a) Invasive melanoma—cutaneous intradermal metastasis (clinical view)

Following excision of a primary melanoma, the tumor can recur as a solitary lesion or as multiple intradermal lesions. Clinically these usually appear as blue nodules. In this case, an intradermal recurrence is seen overlying the primary melanoma excision scar.

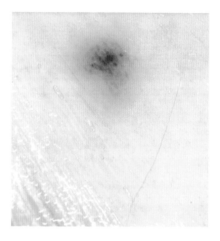

FIGURE 5.78 (b) Invasive melanoma—cutaneous intradermal metastasis (dermoscopy)

Because of the lack of epidermal or junctional pathology, intradermal metastases appear relatively featureless under dermoscopy. This lesion is almost "invisible" when viewed with the surface microscope although it has the most common global pattern of homogeneous pigmentation. Nevertheless, the diagnosis usually relies on clinical suspicion due to their sudden appearance and rapid growth on a background history of primary melanoma.

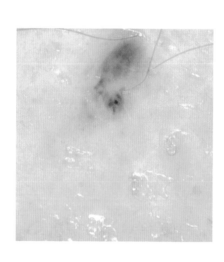

FIGURE 5.79 Invasive melanoma—cutaneous intradermal metastasis (dermoscopy)

The most common dermoscopic color of cutaneous metastases is brown-gray as seen here.

FIGURE 5.80 Invasive melanoma—cutaneous intradermal metastasis (dermoscopy)

Amelanotic or hypomelanotic cutaneous metastases are commonly seen.

FIGURE 5.81 Invasive melanoma—cutaneous metastasis (dermoscopy)*

Here the saccular variant is seen.

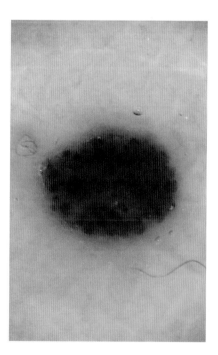

* *This photograph was kindly provided by Dr Riccardo Bono, Rome, Italy.*

FIGURE 5.82 Invasive melanoma—cutaneous metastasis (dermoscopy)†

When vessels are present the most common are polymorphous (more than one type) and winding vessels (resembling a corkscrew) as seen here.

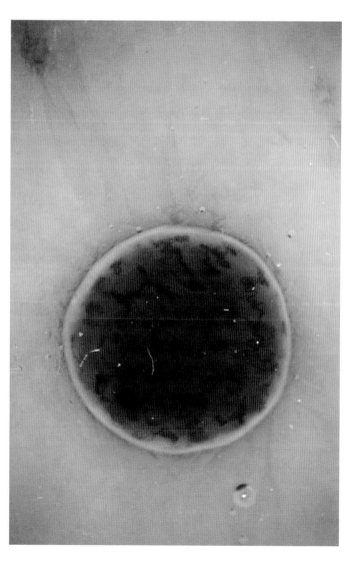

† *This photograph was kindly provided by Dr Riccardo Bono, Rome, Italy.*

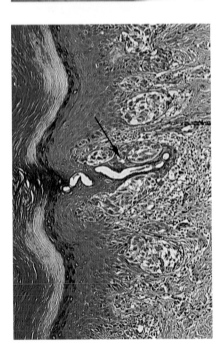

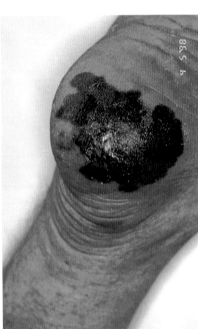

FIGURE 5.83 Acral lentiginous melanoma (histopathology)
In acral lentiginous melanoma there is often hyperplasia of the epidermis with a variable proliferation of atypical melanocytes. In this case there are nests of atypical melanocytes which can also be seen to involve the eccrine (sweat) duct (arrow) as it passes through the epidermis. Notice also the convoluted pattern of the eccrine duct as it passes through the stratum corneum. Magnification ×50 (H & E stain).

FIGURE 5.84 (a) Acral lentiginous melanoma (clinical view)

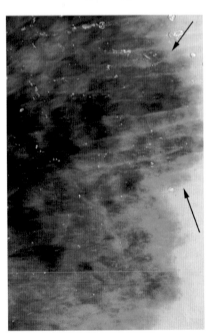

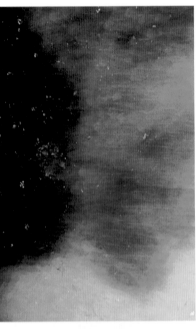

FIGURE 5.84 (b) (i) Acral lentiginous melanoma (dermoscopy)
Melanoma on the palms and soles, like benign nevi, have a different dermoscopy appearance than on non-volar sites. In particular, the macular/ flat (often in situ) component of acral lentiginous melanoma usually has a distinct pigment network called the parallel ridge pattern (arrow). Here the ridges of the surface skin markings (in contrast to the furrows as in Figure 2.11) are predominantly pigmented. The parallel ridge pattern occurs in 86% of acral lentiginous melanomas (2.1 mm Breslow depth).

FIGURE 5.84 (b) (ii) Acral lentiginous melanoma (dermoscopy)
In some of the tumor the macular component loses areas of parallel ridge pattern which is replaced by irregular diffuse pigmentation with variable shades from tan to black. This is also an important diagnostic feature with an 85% sensitivity and 97% specificity for the diagnosis of acral melanoma.

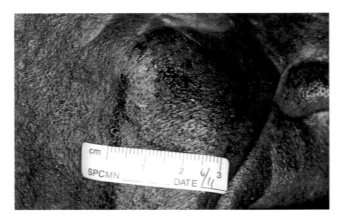

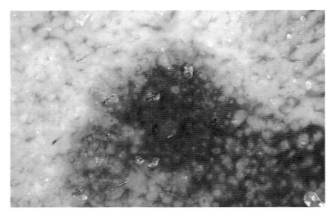

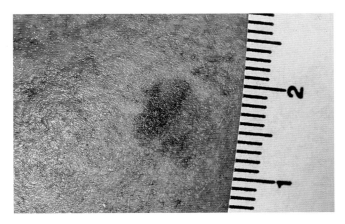

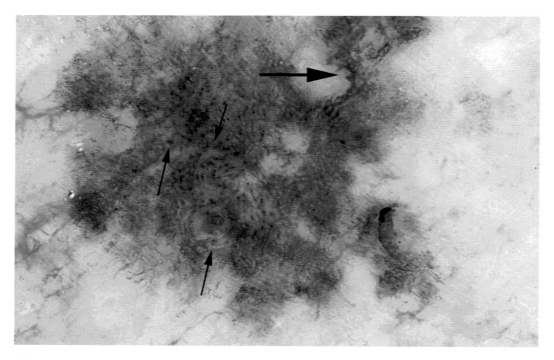

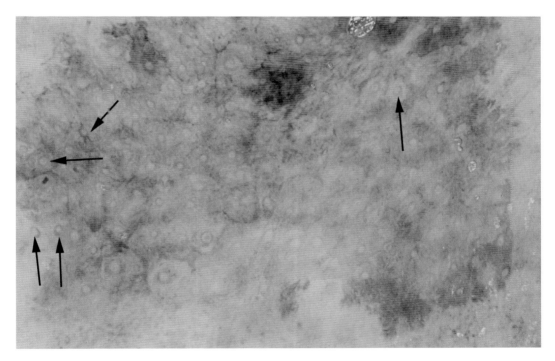

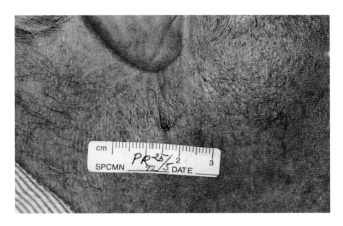

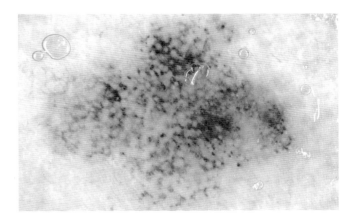

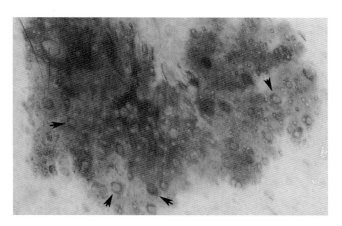

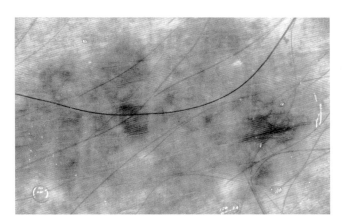

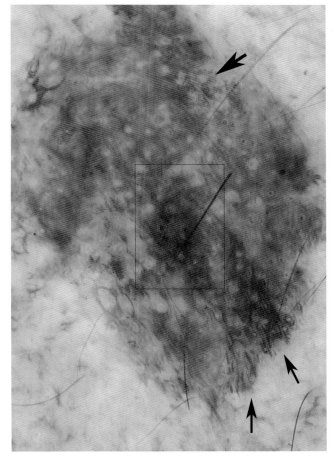

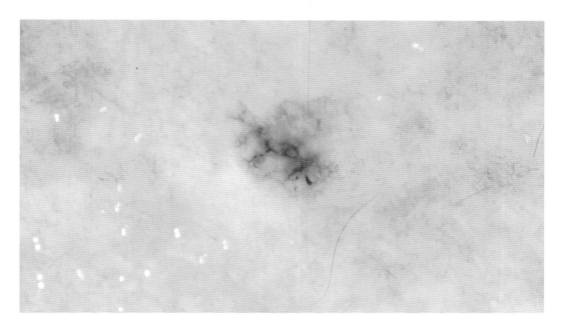

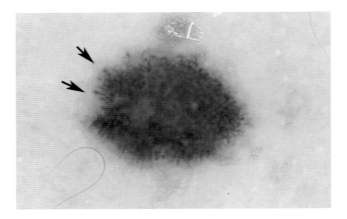

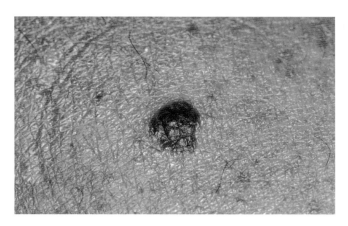

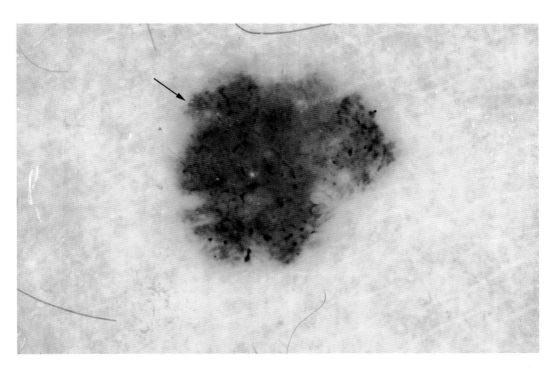

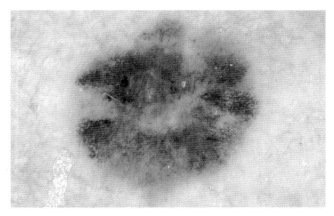

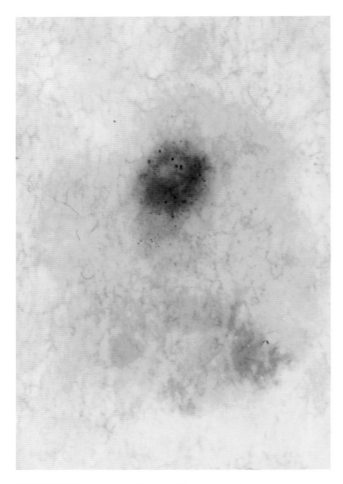

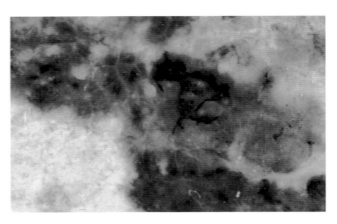

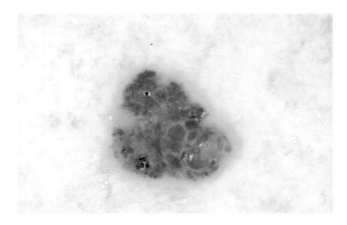

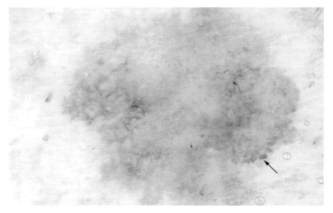

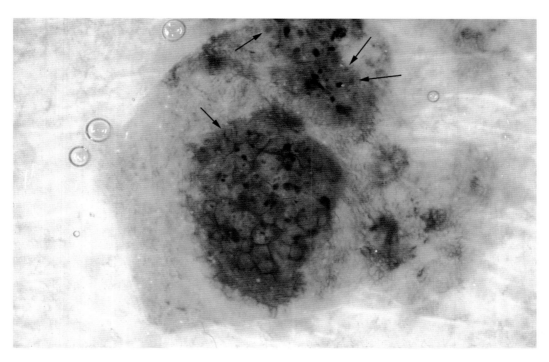

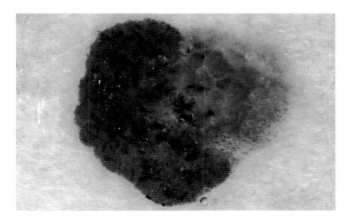

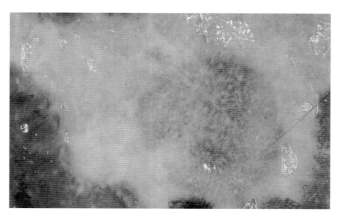

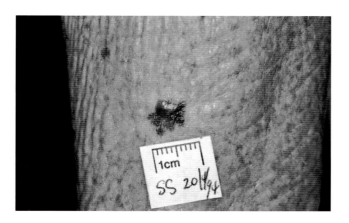

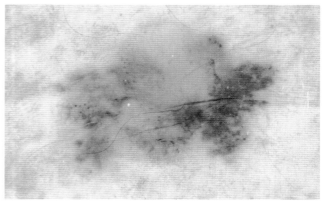

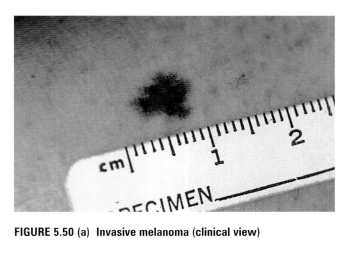

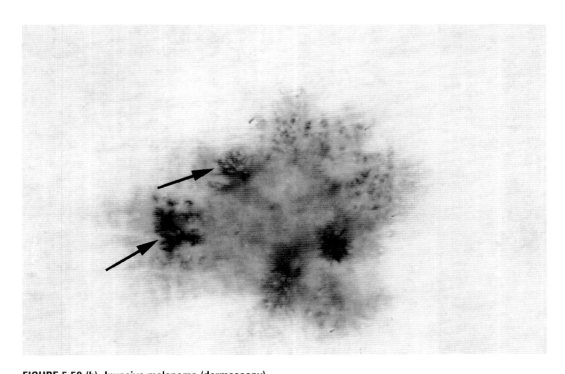

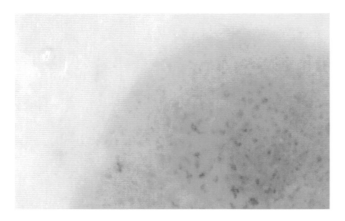

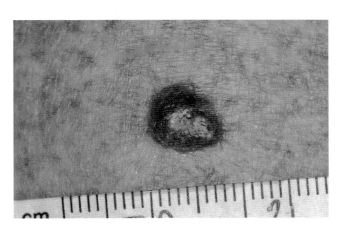

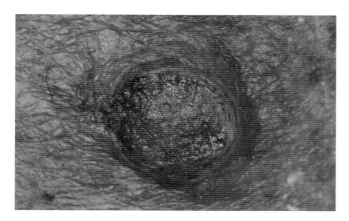

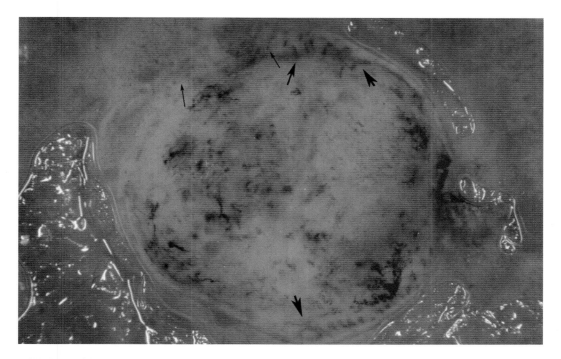

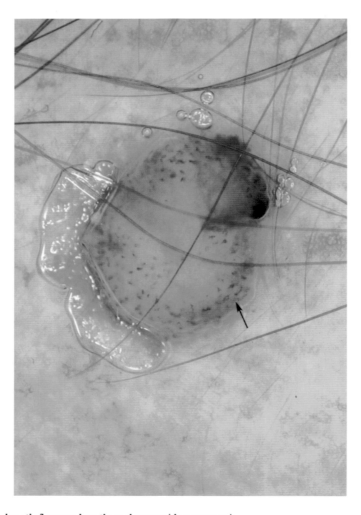

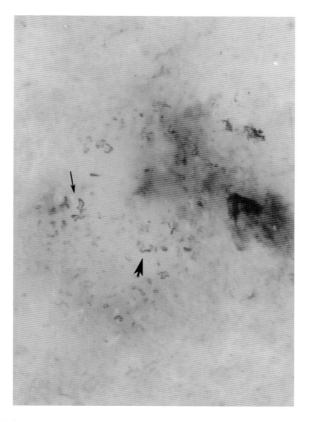

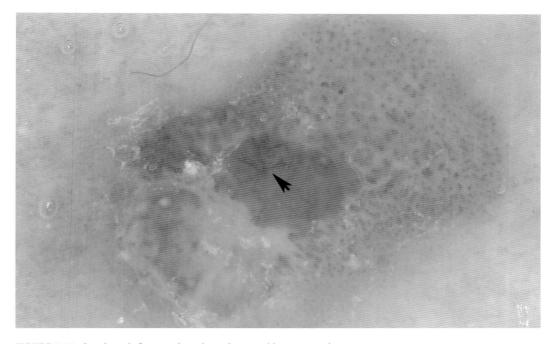

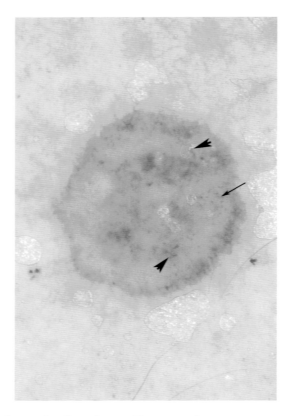

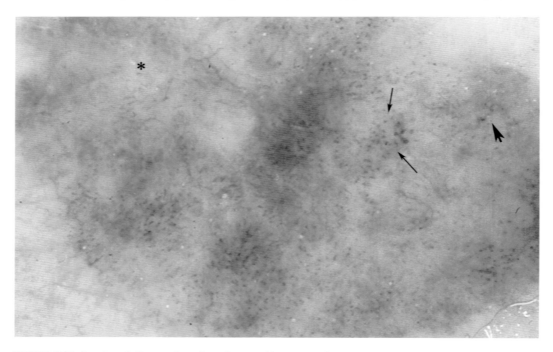

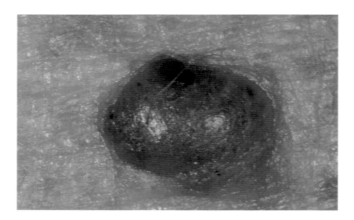

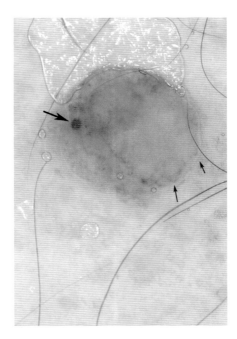

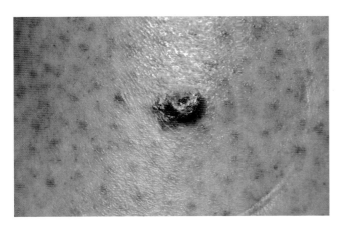

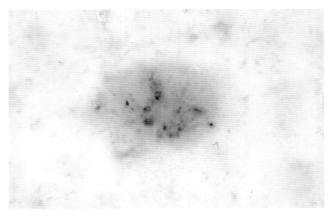

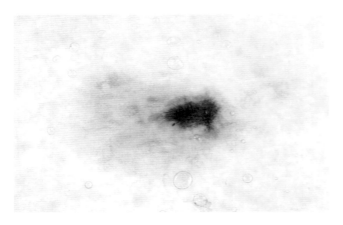

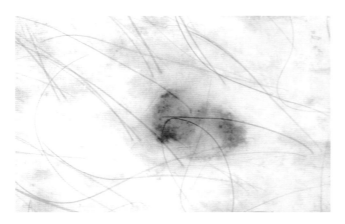

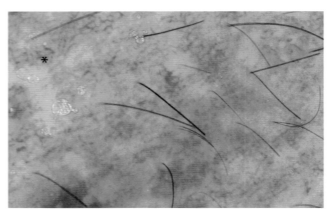

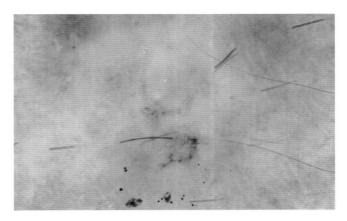

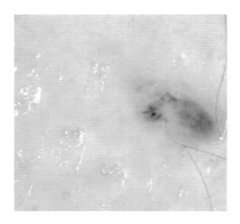

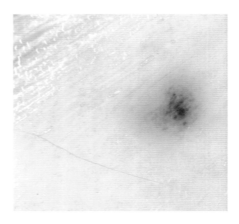

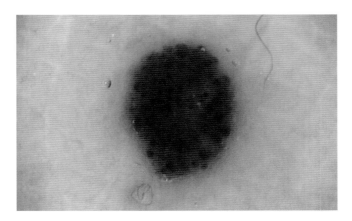

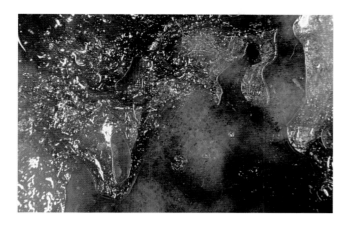

FIGURE 5.84 (b) (iii) Acral lentiginous melanoma (dermoscopy)
The dermoscopic features of the invasive melanoma components of acral lentiginous melanoma become more similar to classical non-volar melanoma as the Breslow depth increases. Here widespread blue-white veil and multiple brown dots are seen.

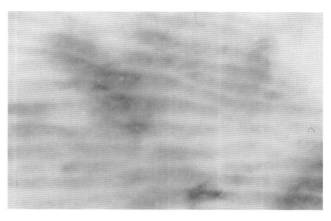

FIGURE 5.85 Acral lentiginous melanoma (dermoscopy)
This lesion has parallel ridge pattern throughout its surface. The parallel ridge pattern has a 99% specificity for the diagnosis of acral melanoma. Diagnosis: In situ melanoma.

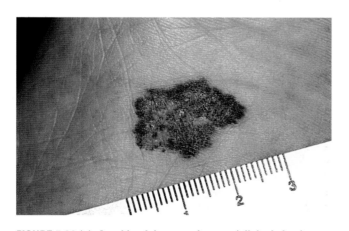

FIGURE 5.86 (a) Acral lentiginous melanoma (clinical view)

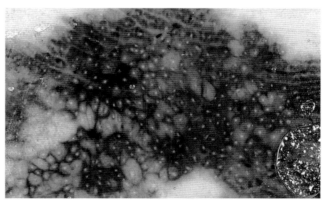

FIGURE 5.86 (b) Acral lentiginous melanoma (dermoscopy)
This asymmetrical lesion has areas of parallel ridge pattern and irregularly distributed black globules. Note the white dots which are the openings of eccrine sweat ducts (0.5 mm Breslow depth).

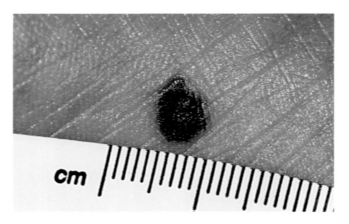

FIGURE 5.87 (a) Acral lentiginous melanoma (clinical view)

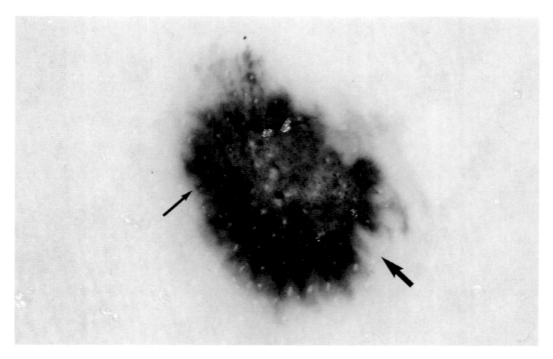

FIGURE 5.87 (b) Acral lentiginous melanoma (dermoscopy)

Subtle remnants of the parallel ridge pattern are seen at the edge of the lesion (large arrow). However in most parts this has been replaced by diffuse dark pigmentation with irregular shades from brown to black. Elsewhere, the lesion has classical features of non-volar melanoma with blue-white veil, multiple brown dots and a pseudopod/radial streaming at the edge of the lesion (small arrow). Again note the white dots of the openings of the eccrine sweat ducts (1.2 mm Breslow depth).

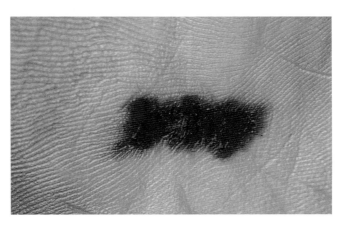

FIGURE 5.88 (a) Acral lentiginous melanoma (clinical view)

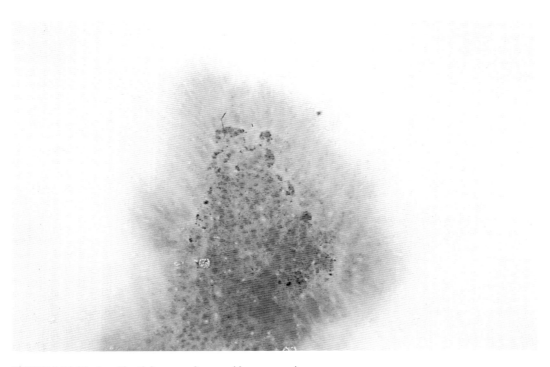

FIGURE 5.88 (b) Acral lentiginous melanoma (dermoscopy)
This lesion shows areas of parallel ridge pattern and diffuse pigmentation in its macular component and multiple brown dots and pinpoint telangiectases more centrally (2.2 mm Breslow depth).

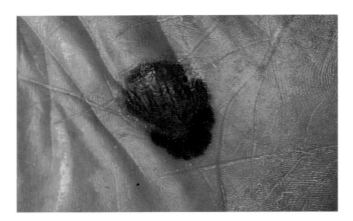

FIGURE 5.89 (a) Acral lentiginous melanoma (clinical view)

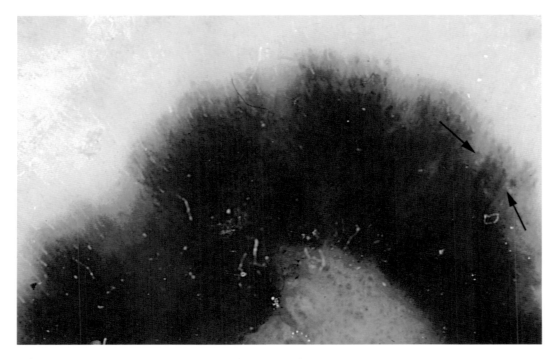

FIGURE 5.89 (b) Acral lentiginous melanoma (dermoscopy)
Only small areas of parallel ridge pattern are seen (delineated by arrows), with the majority replaced by diffuse pigmentation. Note the amelanotic nodule with subtle pinpoint telangiectases. In our experience, amelanotic melanoma is more common on volar sites.

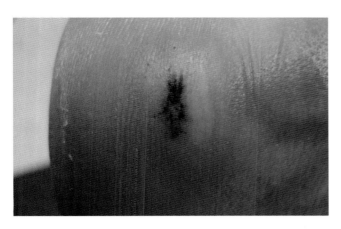

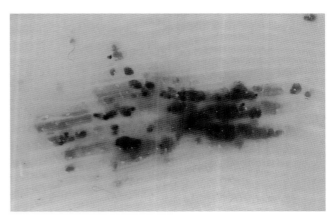

FIGURE 5.90 (a) Talon noir (clinical)

Talon noir (black heel) appears most commonly in athletes and is due to intra-corneal hemorrhage. Clinically it may resemble acral melanoma.

FIGURE 5.90 (b) Talon noir (dermoscopy)

Here the classic dermoscopic features of red-black lacunes overlying the acral ridges ("pebbles on a ridge" pattern) makes the diagnosis certain.

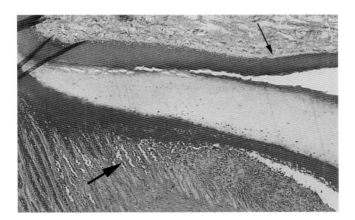

FIGURE 5.91 Subungual melanoma (histopathology)

The melanoma is arising from the nail matrix (large arrow). Immediately above the matrix is the nail plate. The epithelium above the nail plate belongs to the proximal nail fold (small arrow). Magnification ×20 (H & E stain).

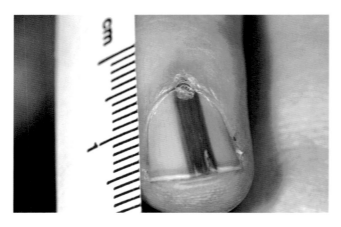

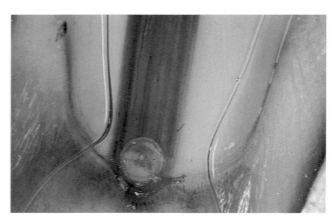

FIGURE 5.92 (a) Subungual melanoma (clinical view)

This lesion has been recently biopsied at the nail matrix and proximal nail fold. Early subungual melanoma commences as a pigmented stripe (longitudinal melanonychia) with an enlarging width.

FIGURE 5.92 (b) Subungual melanoma (dermoscopy)

The presence of brown lines throughout the full length of the nail indicates that the lesion is due to proliferation of melanocytes within the nail matrix (nevus or melanoma). These brown lines are more irregular in width, spacing and parallelism (not all straight) compared with subungal nevi. However, the history of increased width of the longitudinal melanonychia is probably the key to very early diagnosis of subungual melanoma. Diagnosis: In situ melanoma.

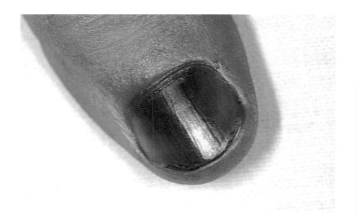

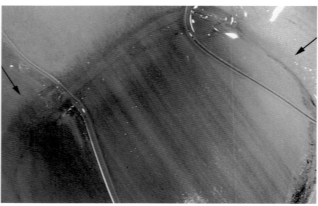

FIGURE 5.93 (a) Subungual melanoma (clinical view)

FIGURE 5.93 (b) Subungual melanoma (dermoscopy)

Here the enlarging pigmented stripe has nearly involved the entire nail plate. Indeed extension of pigmentation has involved the lateral nail fold and one area of and beyond the proximal nail fold (arrows) (i.e. positive Hutchinson's sign) (in situ melanoma).

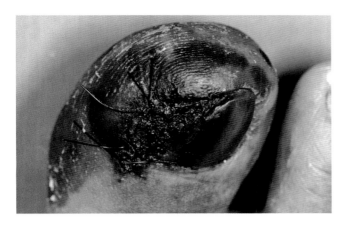

FIGURE 5.94 (a) Subungual melanoma (clinical view)

This melanoma commenced as a subungual lesion. The area of pigmentation later involved the nail folds and surrounding skin (positive Hutchinson's sign). Nail dystrophy and destruction heralds the onset of invasion.

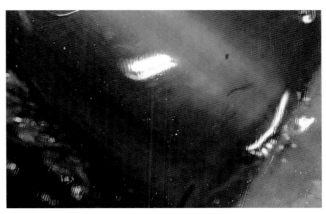

FIGURE 5.94 (b) Subungual melanoma (dermoscopy)

(Melanoma 1.2 mm Breslow depth.)

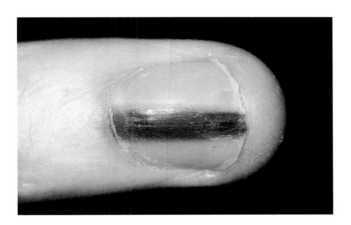

FIGURE 5.95 (a) Subungual melanoma (clinical)[‡]

[‡] *This photograph was kindly provided by Dr Luc Thomas, Lyon, France.*

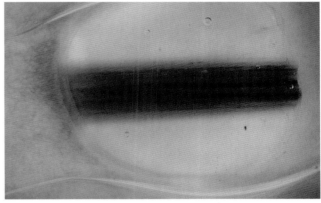

FIGURE 5.95 (b) Subungual melanoma (dermoscopy)[§]

Here the brown lines lack uniformity of width, spacing, and parallelism (with some not straight).

[§] *This photograph was kindly provided by Dr Luc Thomas, Lyon, France.*

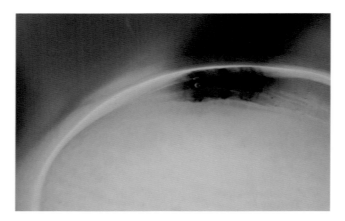

FIGURE 5.95 (c) Subungual melanoma (free edge dermoscopy)[¶]
The position of pigment within the free edge of the nail plate indicates the position of the lesion within the nail matrix; where pigment in the lower half of the nail plate indicating the lesion lies in the distal matrix and pigment in the upper half of the nail plate indicative of a lesion in the proximal matrix. Such an observation allows accurate matrix biopsy, sometimes reducing nail dystrophy (since biopsy of the distal matrix will induce less nail damage). In this case the free edge has pigment in both the upper and lower halves of the nail plate indicating that the biopsy needs to be throughout both the proximal and distal matrix.

[¶] *This photograph was kindly provided by Dr Luc Thomas, Lyon, France.*

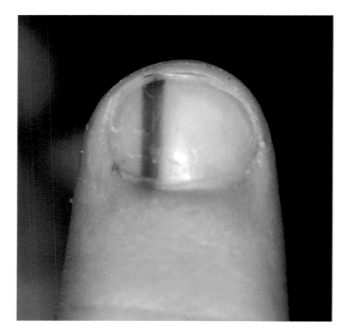

FIGURE 5.96 (a) Subungual nevus (clinical)[**]

[**] *This photograph was kindly provided by Dr Luc Thomas, Lyon, France.*

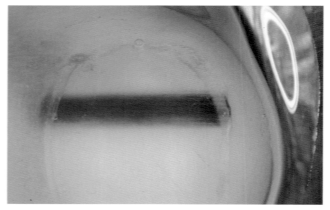

FIGURE 5.96 (b) Subungual nevus (dermoscopy)[††]
Brown lines under dermoscopy indicates the lesion is melanocytic in origin (melanoma or nevus). While nevi tend to have more uniform width, color, spacing, and parallelism of these lines sometimes they can be difficult to discern from early melanoma.

[††] *This photograph was kindly provided by Dr Luc Thomas, Lyon, France.*

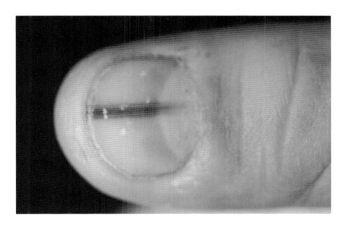

FIGURE 5.97 (a) Subungual nevus (clinical)‡‡

‡‡ *This photograph was kindly provided by Dr Luc Thomas, Lyon, France.*

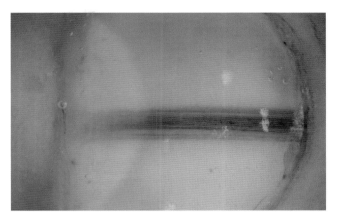

FIGURE 5.97 (b) Subungual nevus (dermoscopy)§§
Here the brown lines are irregular in width and parallelism indicating the need for biopsy.

§§ *Photograph kindly provided by Dr Luc Thomas, Lyon, France.*

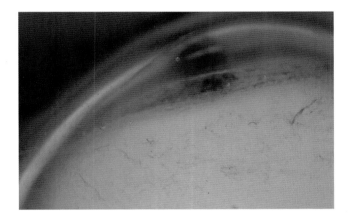

FIGURE 5.97 (c) Subungual nevus (free edge dermoscopy)¶¶
The pigment occupies the lower half of the nail plate free edge indicating the need for biopsy in the distal matrix (avoiding a more destructive result if biopsy of the proximal matrix was required).

¶¶ *This photograph was kindly provided by Dr Luc Thomas, Lyon, France.*

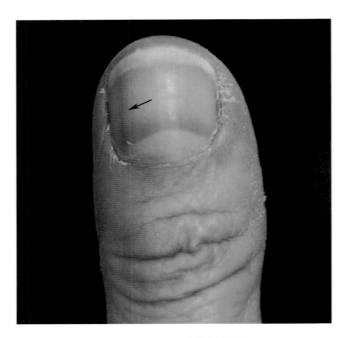

FIGURE 5.98 (a) Subungual lentigo (clinical)∗∗∗

The arrow indicates the area of longitudinal melanonychia.

∗∗∗*This photograph was kindly provided by Dr Luc Thomas, Lyon, France.*

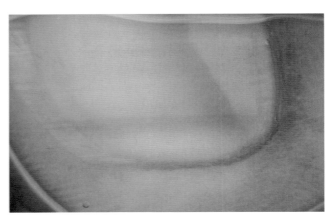

FIGURE 5.98 (b) Subungual lentigo (dermoscopy)†††

Subungual melanotic macules (most commonly due to a lentigo, ethnic (dark skinned races), medications, endocrine disorders, or repetitive trauma) present as longitudinal melanonychia due to increased melanin production without proliferation of nail matrix melanocytes. Most commonly these all present with gray background and fine regular gray lines, as seen here. Subungual lentigo are normally solitary in contrast to the multiple nature of ethnic, endocrine, and drug-induced nail lesions.

††† *This photograph was kindly provided by Dr Luc Thomas, Lyon, France.*

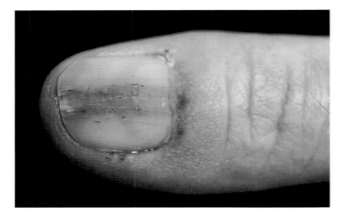

FIGURE 5.99 (a) Subungual melanotic macule—chronic trauma (clinical)‡‡‡

‡‡‡ *This photograph was kindly provided by Dr Luc Thomas, Lyon, France.*

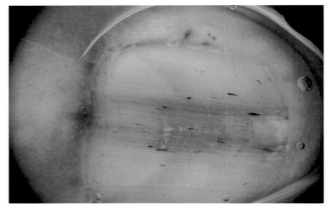

FIGURE 5.99 (b) Subungual melanotic macule—chronic trauma (dermoscopy)§§§

Here repeated trauma causes gray lines with overlying linear hemorrhages.

§§§ *This photograph was kindly provided by Dr Luc Thomas, Lyon, France*

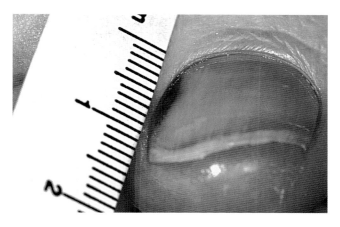

FIGURE 5.100 (a) Subungual hemorrhage (clinical view)

The most common differential diagnosis of subungual melanoma is a subungual hematoma.

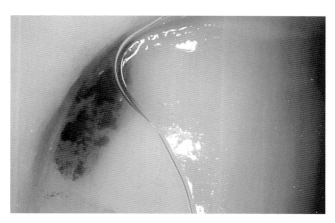

FIGURE 5.100 (b) Subungual hemorrhage (dermoscopy)

Here the distinguishing features are a lack of a melanin (brown) pigment lines throughout the entire length of the nail and large irregular globules of red-blue pigment (blood spots).

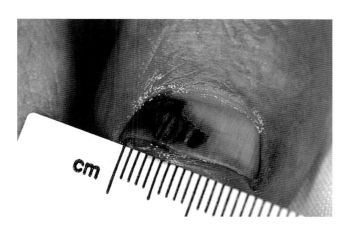

FIGURE 5.101 (a) Subungual hemorrhage (clinical view)

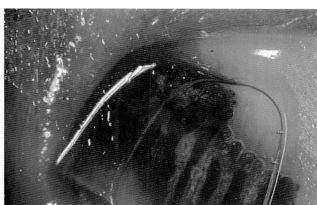

FIGURE 5.101 (b) Subungual hemorrhage (dermoscopy)

Note the area of sparing at the proximal nail fold. In contrast to subungual melanoma, subungual hematomas form an area of sparing of pigmentation at the proximal nail fold as the nail grows out.

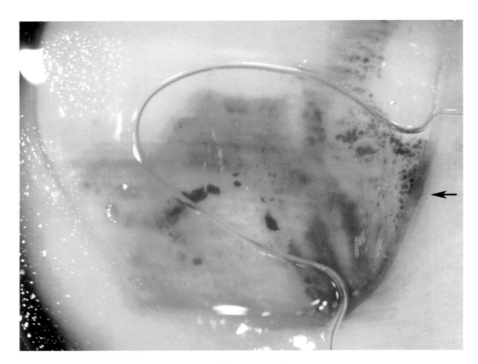

FIGURE 5.102 (a) Subungual hemorrhage (dermoscopy)
While background brown pigmentation can sometimes be seen in subungual hemorrage, brown lines occupying the full length of the nail are never seen. The proximal nail fold (cuticle) is shown for orientation (arrow).

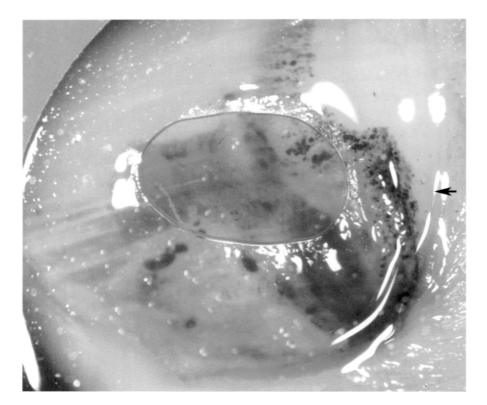

FIGURE 5.102 (b) Subungual hemorrhage (dermoscopy)
This lesion was monitored over 3 months. Note the formation of increasing proximal sparing of pigment from the cuticle occurring as the hemorrhage grows out of the nail. Furthermore the architecture of the pigmentation remains unchanged.

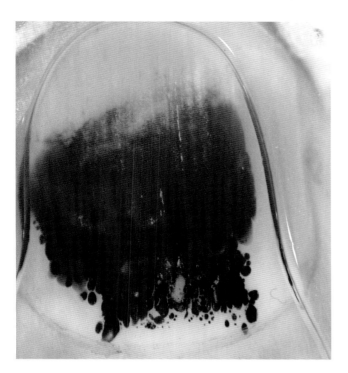

FIGURE 5.103 (a) Subungual hemorrhage—baseline image (dermoscopy)

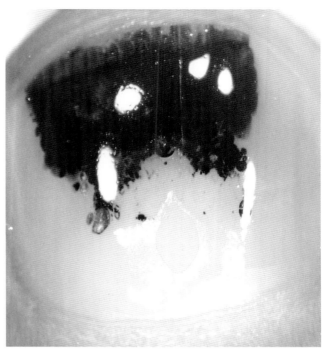

FIGURE 5.103 (b) Subungual hemorrhage—follow-up image (dermoscopy)
Again the hemorrhage grows out of the nail without extension of pigment.

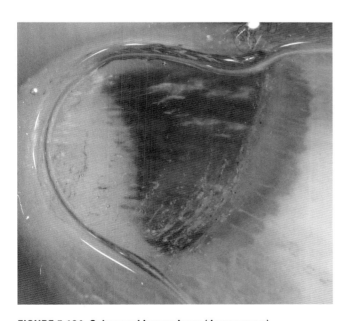

FIGURE 5.104 Subungual hemorrhage (dermoscopy)
Rarely a pseudo-Hutchinson's sign can be found in subungual hemorrhage (as seen here extending from the proximal nail fold).

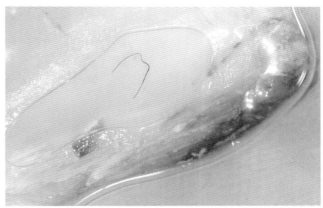

FIGURE 5.105 Subungual infection (dermoscopy)
Subungual infections are characterized by pigment not seen in melanocytic lesions, such as yellow or green. No blood spots or brown lines throughout the length of the nail are seen. In this lesion trichophyton was cultured from nail clippings confirming the diagnosis.

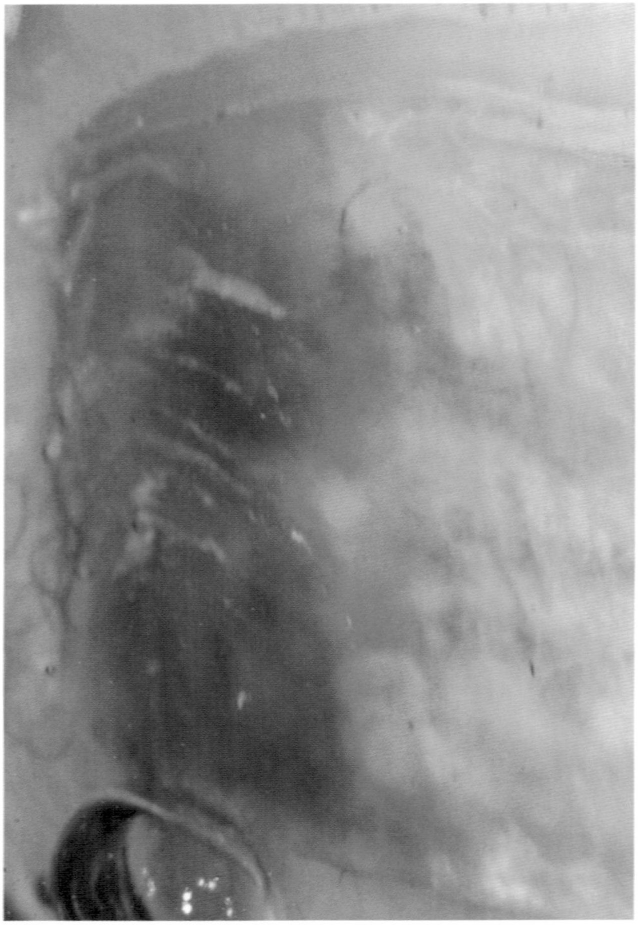

FIGURE 5.106 Subungual infection (dermoscopy)

CHAPTER SIX

NON-MELANOCYTIC PIGMENTED TUMORS

Dermoscopy is particularly helpful in distinguishing non-melanocytic pigmented tumors from melanoma.

Pigmented basal cell carcinoma

The majority of basal cell carcinomas are amelanotic.[1] In contrast to dark skin races where the majority of BCCs are pigmented, only 7% of BCCs are pigmented in anglo-celtic people. Nevertheless, these lesions cause clinical confusion because of their similarity with melanoma. However, under dermoscopy, they are usually easily distinguishable by their features of:

- Negative feature (cannot be found)
  - pigment network
- Positive feature (at least one feature found)
  - ulceration
  - large blue-gray ovoid nests
  - multiple blue-gray globules
  - leaf-like areas
  - spoke wheel areas
  - arborizing (treelike) telangiectasia

This method will allow the diagnosis of 93% of pigmented BCC, with a specificity of 89% for invasive melanoma and 92% for benign pigmented lesions.[1]

Seborrheic keratosis

This common, often pigmented, benign tumor primarily seen in the elderly can vary morphologically from a flat lesion (macule) to a large nodule. Clinically, some pigmented superficial seborrheic keratoses can be difficult to distinguish from the ephelis, lentigo and lentigo maligna melanoma, while larger nodular seborrheic keratoses may be difficult to distinguish from atypical nevi and melanoma. However, perhaps with the exception of the hemangioma, dermoscopy aids in the positive diagnosis of the seborrheic keratosis more than any other lesion. Its major features are[2–4]:

- fissures/ridges (common)
- crypts (common)
- multiple milia-like cysts (common)
- well demarcated border (common)
- keratin (some)
- absent network (majority)
- fingerprint-like areas (some)
- fat fingers (some)
- moth-eaten edge (some)
- multiple blue-gray globules (rare variant)
- regularly arranged loops of hairpin vessels often with surrounding white halos (some)

The latter feature is seen particularly in irritated seborrheic keratoses. While network-like structures can occur in seborrheic keratoses, these are usually psuedo-networks presenting as a variant of fissures and ridges or fingerprint-like areas.[3] However, 7% of seborrheic keratoses may have areas of a pigment network not distinguishable from melanocytic lesions.[4] While multiple small milia-like cysts can be seen in compound nevi and seborrheic keratoses, multiple *large* milia-like cysts are virtually pathognomonic for the latter diagnosis. Finally, it should be emphasized that milia-like cysts and crypts may not be visualized with cross-polarized surface microscopes (see Figure 1.8).

The dermoscopic features of the more rare **verrucous epidermal nevus** overlap with the seborrheic keratosis.

Hemangioma

The majority of lesions referred to as hemangiomas are hamartomas composed of capillary vessels (capillary hemangioma), large vascular spaces (cavernous hemangioma), or a mixture of both. Because histologically they often contain mixed elements of capillary and cavernous spaces, the authors have not differentiated between the two sub-types. Angiokeratoma is included within the diagnosis of hemangioma.[5] The dermoscopic features of hemangiomas are:

- red-blue color (universal)
- red-blue lacunes (majority)
- red-blue as the solitary color (majority)
- dark to black lacunes (some)
- peripheral erythema (some)
- hemorrhagic crust (some)
- scar-like depigmentation (some)

Dark to black lacunes are found in angiokeratoma or thrombosed hemangioma.[5] Blue-white veil-like areas are seen in many hemangioma. However, true blue-white veil can never be diagnosed in the presence of red-blue lacunes. Hence, hemangiomas are usually very easily distinguished from melanoma.

Dermatofibroma

Dermatofibromas (histiocytomas, sclerosing hemangioma) are common lesions found frequently on the lower limbs. In contrast to the clinical findings of hard, usually brown nodules that characteristically dimple when pressed at the edges (positive pinch sign), the dermoscopic findings may mimic those of a melanocytic lesion. In particular the variable epidermal changes of lichenification, atrophy, and basal proliferation and pigmentation lead to variable and subtle dermoscopic features, which overlap with melanocytic-derived lesions (such as the presence of a delicate network).

The dermoscopic features of dermatofibroma[6–9] are:

- delicate (fine) discrete network (common)
- white scar-like patch (common)
- white network (some)
- homogenous brown or red-blue pigmentation (some)
- erythema (some)
- dotted vessels (some)
- brown globule-like structures (some)

Usually the network is found at the periphery, but in some cases it can be found throughout the lesion. In contrast, the white scar-like patch is usually found centrally, but can occur throughout the lesion or be multifocal.[6] Often perifollicular depigmentation may lead to the impression of a multifocal scarring. A variant of the white scar-like patch is the white network. It too is usually central in position. The cords of the white network are usually thicker than the negative network seen in some melanocytic lesions, however sometimes the morphology can be similar. Brown globule-like structures

can occur in some lesions. However, these are often ring-like structures derived from the pigment network or small crypts rather than true brown globules seen in melanocytic lesions.

The most common dermoscopic global pattern of dermatofibromas is a fine discrete network with a central scar-like white patch. Ninety-four percent of dermatofibromas have combinations of the basic morphological structures of fine discrete network, white scar-like patch, white network, and homogeneous brown or red-blue pigmentation.[6] Like most lesions, dermatofibromas have a different appearance under cross-polarized surface microscopes. In particular, erythema and vascular structures are more prominent with non-contact cross polarization and the white scar-like patch seen with the liquid glass plate devices may appear as "white streaks".[7]

Lichen planus-like keratosis (lichenoid keratosis)

Lichen planus-like keratoses are thought to be regressing seborrheic keratoses or solar lentigo. They are most commonly seen as single lesions on the upper extremities, face, and chest.[10] They usually have the history of a preceding pigmented macule/plaque (solar lentigo or seborrheic keratosis), are often rapidly changing, and many are pruritic (with a range of other abnormal sensations). In the early phase (over weeks to months) they present as either an erythematous or violaceous plaque. Following this they flatten and are often seen clinically as gray macules. The dermoscopic features of this lesion[11–13] usually reflect their aetiology:

- diffuse multiple blue-gray dots (common)
- localized multiple blue-gray dots (common)
- areas of uniform tan pigmentation (common)
- absent brown globules (common)
- areas of seborrheic keratosis or solar lentigo (some)

Since solar lentigo may have a fine pigment network (see Chapter 3), some cases of lichen planus-like keratoses (that represent regressing solar lentigo) can be difficult to distinguish from lentigo maligna or regressing melanoma. In such cases the presence of brown finger print-like areas in addition to a fine network favors the diagnosis of lichen planus-like keratosis. Finally, when melanophages (multiple blue/gray dots) appear high in the papillary dermis in these lesions they may have a gray/brown color.

Bowen's disease
(in situ squamous cell carcinoma)

In anglo-celtic races Bowen's disease presents as a scaly erythematous macule or plaque on sun-exposed sites. Much less commonly Bowen's may be pigmented. The dermoscopic features of Bowen's disease are[14]:

- Glomerular vessels (common)
- Scale (common)
- Dotted vessels (some)
- Homogeneous brown pigmentation (common in pigmented variant)
- Brown globules (common in pigmented variant)

Since dotted vessels, homogeneous brown pigmentation, and irregularly distributed brown globules may also be a dermoscopy presentation of light colored melanoma, biopsy of pigmented Bowen's before treatment is essential. Finally, the dermoscopic features of plaque psoriasis overlap substantially with non-pigmented Bowen's disease[15]. However, the multiple nature and distribution of psoriatic plaques usually enables distinction between the two entities.

Clear cell acanthoma

Clear cell acanthomas are benign epidermal tumors characterized histopathologically by the presence of glycogen filled "clear" keratinocytes. They usually present as solitary, slowly growing pink or red dome-shaped nodules, and are most commonly found on the lower legs of middle-aged or elderly people.[16] While these lesions are non-pigmented, because of their characteristic dermoscopic features they are included in this chapter. The dermoscopic features of clear cell acanthomas are enlarged dotted/glomerular vessels in a reticular/linear or so-called "string of pearls" pattern. A variant of this pattern can also be seen in plaque psoriasis.[15-20]

References

1. Menzies, S, Westerhoff, K, Rabinovitz, H, Kopf, A, McCarthy, W, Katz, B. The surface microscopy of pigmented basal cell carcinoma. *Arch Dermatol* 2000; 136: 1012–16.
2. Kopf, AW, Rabinovitz, H, Marghoob, A, et al. "Fat fingers:" a clue in the dermoscopic diagnosis of seborrheic keratoses. *J Am Acad Dermatol* 2006; 55: 1089–91.
3. Braun, RP, Rabinovitz, HS, Krischer, J, et al. Dermoscopy of pigmented seborrheic keratosis: a morphological study. *Arch Dermatol* 2002; 138: 1556–60.
4. De Giorgi, V, Massi, D, Stante, M, Carli, P. False "melanocytic" parameters shown by pigmented seborrheic keratoses: a finding which is not uncommon in dermoscopy. *Dermatol Surg* 2002; 28: 776–9.
5. Zaballos, P, Daufí, C, Puig, S, et al. Dermoscopy of solitary angiokeratomas: a morphological study. *Arch Dermatol* 2007; 143: 318–25.
6. Zaballos, P, Puig, S, Llambrich, A, Malvehy, J. Dermoscopy of dermatofibromas: a prospective morphological study of 412 cases. *Arch Dermatol* 2008; 144: 75–83.
7. Agero, AL, Taliercio, S, Dusza, SW, Salaro, C, Chu, P, Marghoob, AA. Conventional and polarized dermoscopy features of dermatofibroma. *Arch Dermatol* 2006; 142: 1431–7.
8. Arpaia, N, Cassano, N, Vena, GA. Dermoscopic patterns of dermatofibroma. *Dermatol Surg* 2005; 31: 1336–9.
9. Ferrari, A, Soyer, HP, Peris, K, et al. Central white scarlike patch: a dermatoscopic clue for the diagnosis of dermatofibroma. *J Am Acad Dermatol* 2000; 43: 1123–5.
10. Laur, W, Posy, R, Waller, J. Lichen planus-like keratosis. *J Am Acad Dermatol* 1981; 4: 329–36.
11. Bugatti, L, Filosa, G. Dermoscopy of lichen planus-like keratosis: a model of inflammatory regression. *J Eur Acad Dermatol Venereol* 2007; 21: 1392–7.
12. Zaballos, P, Blazquez, S, Puig, S, et al. Dermoscopic pattern of intermediate stage in seborrhoeic keratosis regressing to lichenoid keratosis: report of 24 cases. *Br J Dermatol* 2007; 157: 266–72.
13. Elgart, GW. Seborrheic keratoses, solar lentigines, and lichenoid keratoses. Dermatoscopic features and correlation to histology and clinical signs. *Dermatol Clin* 2001; 19: 347–57.
14. Zalaudek, I, Argenziano, G, Leinweber, B, et al. Dermoscopy of Bowen's disease. *Br J Dermatol* 2004; 150: 1112–6.
15. Vázquez-López, F, Zaballos, P, Fueyo-Casado, A, Sánchez-Martín, J. A dermoscopy subpattern of plaque-type psoriasis: red globular rings. *Arch Dermatol* 2007; 143: 1612.
16. LeBoit, P, Burg, G, Weedon, D, Sarasin, A (eds). *Pathology and Genetics of Skin Tumours*. IARC Press, Lyon, 2006.

17. Bugatti, L, Filosa, G, Broganelli, P, Tomasini, C. Psoriasis-like dermoscopic pattern of clear cell acanthoma. *J Eur Acad Dermatol Venereol* 2003; 17: 452–5.

18. Zalaudek, I, Hofmann-Wellenhof, R, Argenziano, G. Dermoscopy of clear-cell acanthoma differs from dermoscopy of psoriasis. *Dermatology* 2003; 207: 428.

19. Vázquez-López, F, Zaballos, P, Fueyo-Casado, A, Sánchez-Martín, J. A dermoscopy subpattern of plaque-type psoriasis: red globular rings. *Arch Dermatol* 2007; 143: 1612.

20. Blum, A, Metzler, G, Bauer, J, Rassner, G, Garbe, C. The dermatoscopic pattern of clear-cell acanthoma resembles psoriasis vulgaris. *Dermatology* 2001; 203: 50–2.

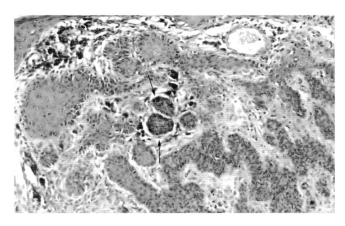

FIGURE 6.1 Pigmented basal cell carcinoma (histopathology)
This section shows a basal cell carcinoma composed of nests of hyperchromatic cells with peripheral palisading. In some cases melanocytes are present within the tumor, causing pigmentation of the tumor nests (arrows). Magnification ×50 (H & E stain).

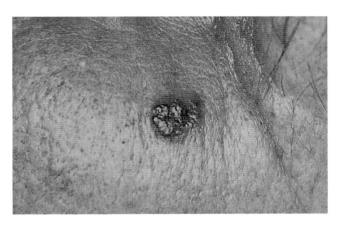

FIGURE 6.2 (a) Pigmented basal cell carcinoma (clinical view)
The majority of BCCs are amelanotic. However, some have significant areas of pigmentation, which can lead to clinical confusion with melanoma.

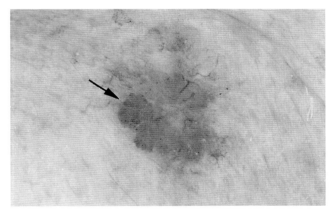

FIGURE 6.2 (b) Pigmented basal cell carcinoma (dermoscopy)
This lesion has an absent pigment network and the positive features of leaf-like areas (arrow), arborizing telangiectases (tree-like with distinct branching) and a large blue-gray ovoid nest (inferior right pole).

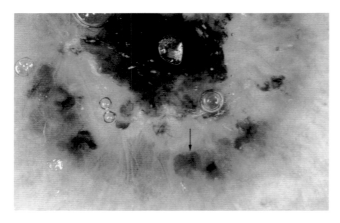

FIGURE 6.3 Pigmented basal cell carcinoma (dermoscopy)
Leaf-like areas (arrow) are discrete structures that usually do not arise from a confluent pigmented tumor body and never from a network. Therefore, they can be easily distinguished from pseudopods found in melanoma. Note the ulceration which is seen in 27% of pigmented BCCs.

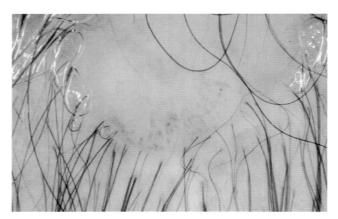

FIGURE 6.4 Pigmented basal cell carcinoma (dermoscopy)
A specific feature of pigmented BCCs (27% sensitivity) is areas of multiple blue-gray globules usually not connected to a pigmented tumor body.

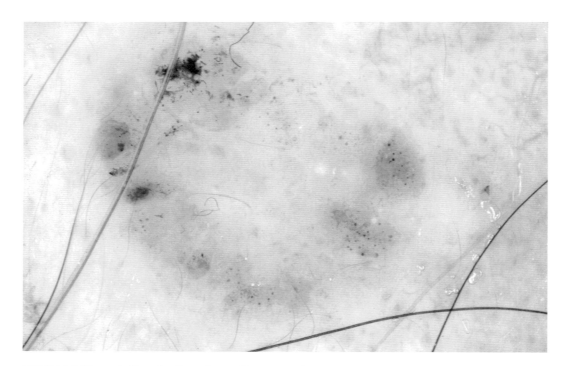

FIGURE 6.5 Pigmented basal cell carcinoma (dermoscopy)
This lesion has an absent pigment network and the positive features of ulceration and multiple blue-gray globules. Multiple blue-gray globules are morphologically different to multiple blue-gray dots (melanophages) because of the former's more distinct and usually larger structures that lack the fine "pepper-like" pattern of multiple blue-gray dots.

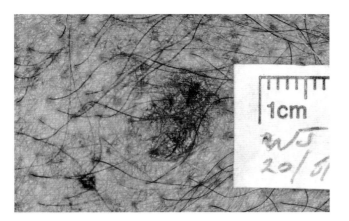

FIGURE 6.6 (a) Pigmented basal cell carcinoma (clinical view)

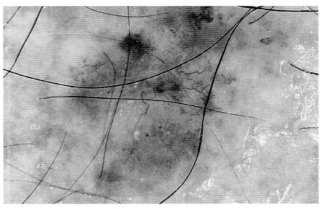

FIGURE 6.6 (b) Pigmented basal cell carcinoma (dermoscopy)
This lesion has an absent network and the positive features of multiple blue-gray globules, arborizing telangiectases and ulceration. Note the milia-like cyst that can be seen in 10% of pigmented BCCs.

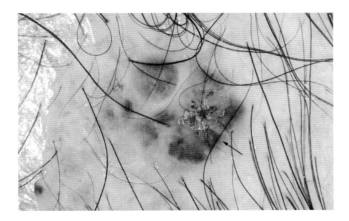

FIGURE 6.7 Pigmented basal cell carcinoma (dermoscopy)
Areas resembling blue-white veil can be seen. However, note the discrete shape of those areas compared with the indistinct and irregular shape of blue-white veil in melanoma. The presence of leaf-like areas (arrow), large blue-gray ovoid nests and absent network confirms the diagnosis of pigmented BCC.

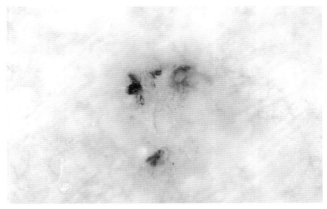

FIGURE 6.8 Pigmented basal cell carcinoma (dermoscopy)
This lesion has an absent network and the positive features of large blue-gray ovoid nests (seen as the single structure at the superior left edge of the lesion), small areas of ulceration, arborizing telangiectases and an atypical leaf-like area near the inferior edge of the lesion. The atypical leaf-like area seen here should not be confused with pseudopods in melanoma because of their lack of connection with a confluent pigmented tumor body or network.

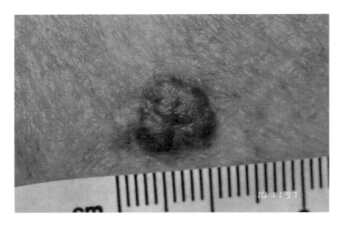

FIGURE 6.9 (a) Pigmented basal cell carcinoma (clinical view)

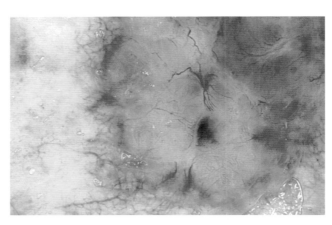

FIGURE 6.9 (b) Pigmented basal cell carcinoma (dermoscopy)
The absent pigment network with arborizing telangiectasia and a solitary large blue-gray ovoid nest define this lesion. Large blue-gray ovoid nests are the most common of the specific positive features of pigmented BCC, with 55% of lesions having them.

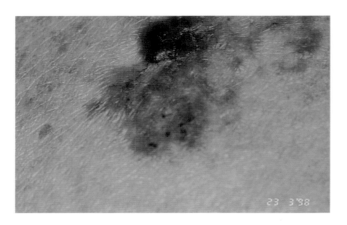

FIGURE 6.10 (a) Pigmented basal cell carcinoma (clinical view)

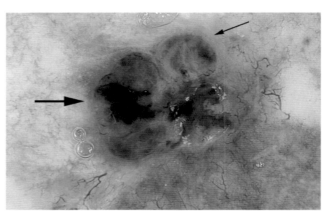

FIGURE 6.10 (b) Pigmented basal cell carcinoma (dermoscopy)
Absent pigment network with arborizing telangiectasia, large blue-gray ovoid nest (small arrow), ulceration and leaf-like area (large arrow) define this lesion.

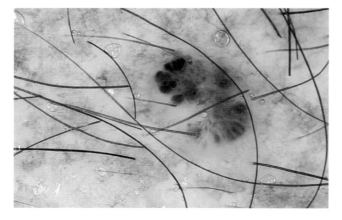

FIGURE 6.11 Pigmented basal cell carcinoma (dermoscopy)
Classical leaf-like areas are seen here. While they are virtually pathognomonic for pigmented BCC (specificity 100%) they only occur in 17% of lesions.

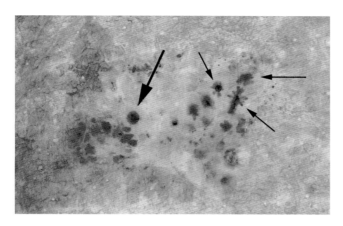

FIGURE 6.12 Pigmented basal cell carcinoma (dermoscopy)
Spoke wheel areas (small arrows) are the least common (10%) of the specific positive features of pigmented BCC. However, like leaf-like areas, they are pathognomonic for pigmented BCC (specificity 100%). Here they have the common morphology of a darkened central axis. In other areas large blue-gray ovoic nests are seen (large arrow). Also found are pigmented nests intermediate between spoke wheel areas and large blue-gray ovoid nests. These have a central dark axis with surrounding irregular brown halos.

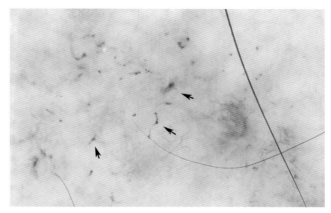

FIGURE 6.13 Pigmented basal cell carcinoma (dermoscopy)
In this lesion a variant of spoke wheel areas are seen (arrows).

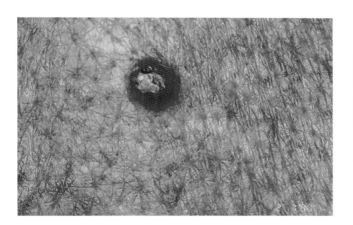

FIGURE 6.14 (a) Pigmented basal cell carcinoma (clinical view)

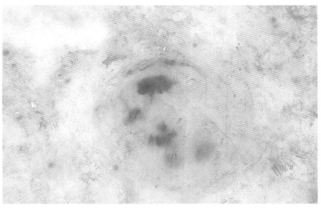

FIGURE 6.14 (b) Pigmented basal cell carcinoma (dermoscopy)
A less common presentation of pigmented BCC is of an amelanotic nodule with red-blue lacunes. These differ from hemangiomas because they are usually sparse in distribution, rather than occupying most of the lesion (see Figures 6.41–6.45).

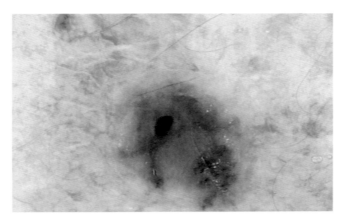

FIGURE 6.15 Pigmented basal cell carcinoma (dermoscopy)

Only 7% of pigmented BCC in white skin races have greater than 75% of their surface area pigmented. In this rare example, the entire area is pigmented.

FIGURE 6.16 Pigmented basal cell carcinoma (dermoscopy)

Only small amounts of pigment (blue-gray globules) are seen in this common presentation of pigmented BCC. 41% of pigmented BCC have less than 25% of their surface pigmented.

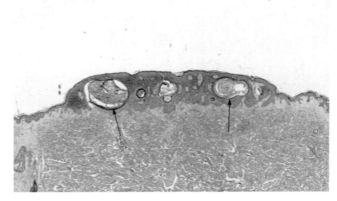

FIGURE 6.17 Seborrheic keratosis (histopathology)

This seborrheic keratosis shows a well-demarcated, epidermally derived lesion composed of small basaloid cells. There is excess keratin production on the surface of the lesion (hyperkeratosis) and small keratin-filled cysts (horn cysts) (arrows). The cells in a seborrheic keratosis may be pigmented. Magnification ×8 (H & E stain).

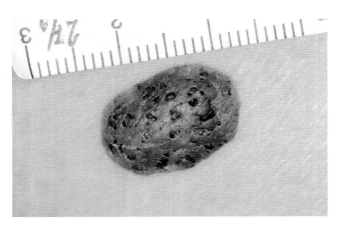

FIGURE 6.18 (a) Seborrheic keratosis (clinical view)
In its classical form the seborrheic keratosis is easily clinically diagnosed by its sharp demarcated "stuck on" appearance and macroscopic crypts or fissures.

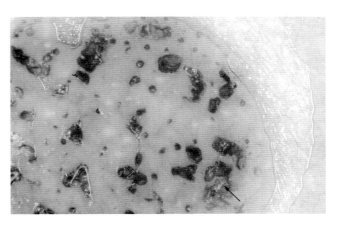

FIGURE 6.18 (b) Seborrheic keratosis (dermoscopy)
The white and yellow multiple milia-like cysts, irregularly shaped crypts, keratin (arrow) and absent network make the diagnosis of seborrheic keratosis certain.

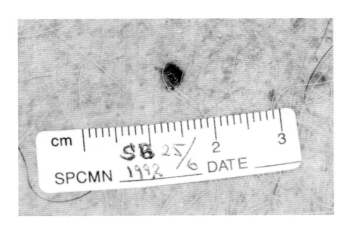

FIGURE 6.19 (a) Seborrheic keratosis (clinical view)
Clinically, some pigmented, superficial seborrheic keratoses can be difficult to distinguish from the lentigo and lentigo maligna melanoma, and larger nodular seborrheic keratoses can be difficult to distinguish from atypical nevi and melanoma.

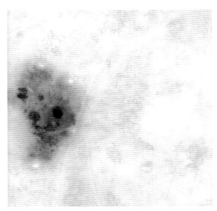

FIGURE 6.19 (b) Seborrheic keratosis (dermoscopy)
Again, the presence of irregular crypts, milia cysts and absent network confirms the diagnosis.

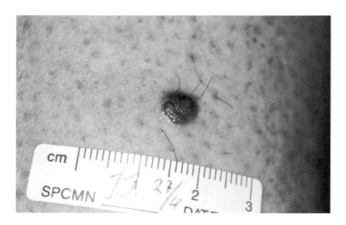

FIGURE 6.20 (a) Seborrheic keratosis (clinical view)

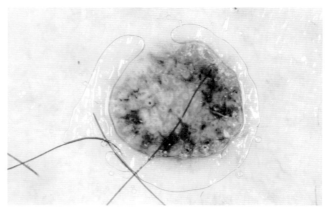

FIGURE 6.20 (b) Seborrheic keratosis (dermoscopy)
The features of this lesion are fissures/ridges, keratin (seen at the periphery of the lesion), regularly arranged loops of telangiectases surrounded by white halos and absent network.

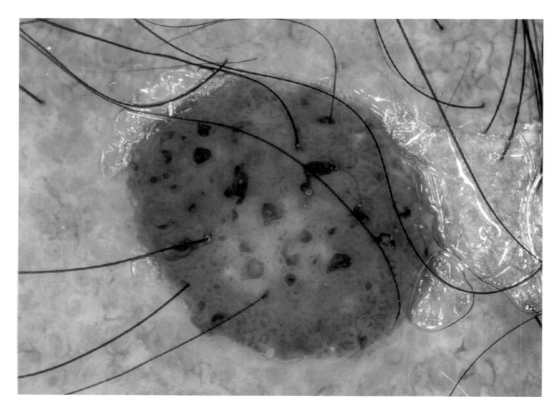

FIGURE 6.21 Seborrheic keratosis (dermoscopy)
Typically, hairpin vessels seen at the periphery of this irritated seborrheic keratoses are more regularly distributed compared with those found in melanoma.

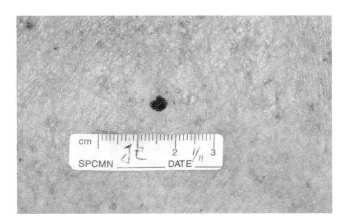

FIGURE 6.22 (a) **Seborrheic keratosis (clinical view)**

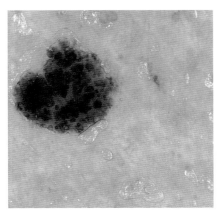

FIGURE 6.22 (b) **Seborrheic keratosis (dermoscopy)**
Like all pigmented lesions in dermoscopy, not all seborrheic keratoses have more than one of the characteristic features of that lesion. Here, the presence of multiple irregular crypts and absent network is all that is required to make the diagnosis.

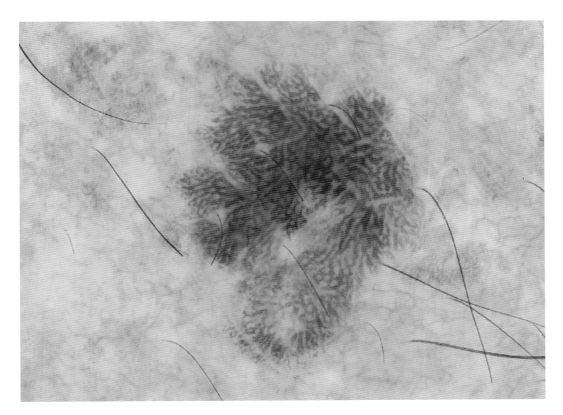

FIGURE 6.23 **Seborrheic keratosis (dermoscopy)**
This lesion has the characteristic pattern of fissures (light areas) and ridges (dark cords).

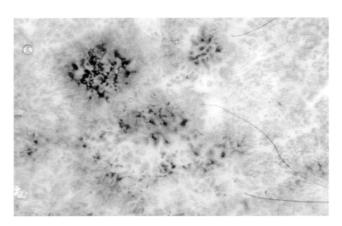

FIGURE 6.24 Seborrheic keratosis (dermoscopy)
Sometimes thicker ridges can form "fat fingers" (arrow).

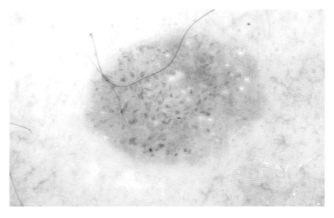

FIGURE 6.25 Seborrheic keratosis (dermoscopy)
Multiple indistinct, light fissures make up this flat seborrheic keratosis.

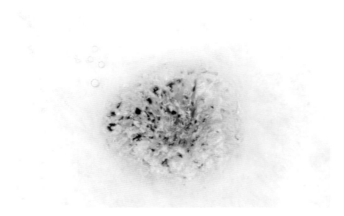

FIGURE 6.26 Seborrheic keratosis (dermoscopy)
Seborrheic keratoses can have varying amounts of focally accumulated keratin—from none to diffusely hyperkeratinized areas, as seen in this lesion.

FIGURE 6.27 Seborrheic keratosis (dermoscopy)
Multiple loops of regularly arranged telangiectases are seen in many irritated seborrheic keratoses. Note the *multiple large* white milia cysts, which are almost pathognomonic for seborrheic keratoses.

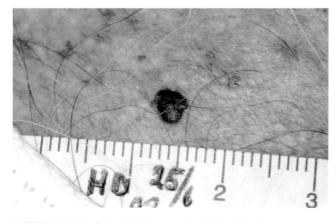

FIGURE 6.28 (a) Seborrheic keratosis (clinical view)
This black nodule gives rise to the suspicion that this lesion is a melanoma.

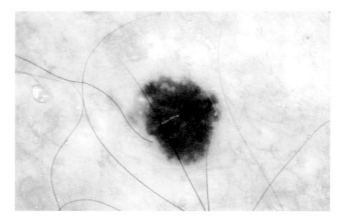

FIGURE 6.28 (b) Seborrheic keratosis (dermoscopy)
However, under dermoscopy it lacks any of the positive features of invasive melanoma and lacks a network. The lesion has the characteristic well-defined border with moth-eaten areas and has a focus of milia cysts.

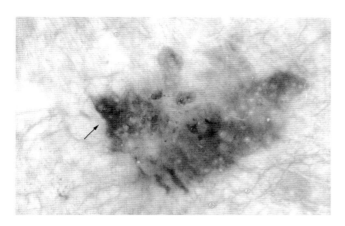

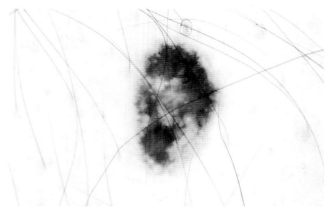

FIGURE 6.29 Seborrheic keratosis (dermoscopy)
The impression of a network is seen (arrow) in this seborrheic keratosis. This "false network" is due to the relative absence of pigment in the crypts and milia cysts that make up the holes of the net. It should be distinguished from the true pigmented network seen in melanocytic-derived lesions. Again note the focus of multiple milia-like cysts. While milia can be present in melanoma, they are usually solitary or scattered sparsely. Finally, note the areas of moth-eaten border particularly at the superior left edge.

FIGURE 6.30 Seborrheic keratosis (dermoscopy)
While the majority of seborrheic keratoses have no true network, a small percentage do. Here, a definite pigment network is seen at the periphery of the lesion, making the diagnosis difficult.

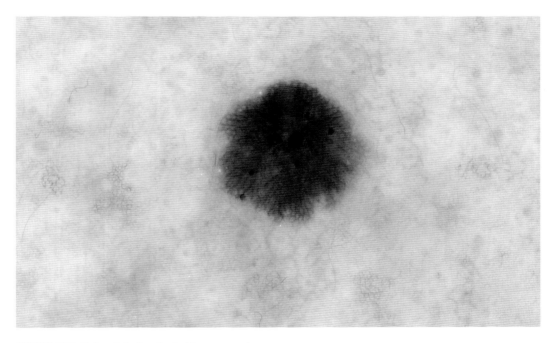

FIGURE 6.31 Seborrheic keratosis (dermoscopy)
While this lesion has a few small milia-like cysts and crypts, it has a distinct pigment network mimicking a melanocytic lesion. However, seborrheic keratoses presenting with such widespread distinct pigment network are uncommon.

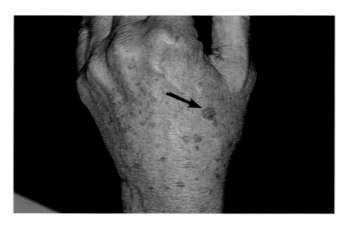

FIGURE 6.32 (a) Seborrheic keratosis (clinical view)
The diagnosis of relatively flat seborrheic keratoses can be difficult.

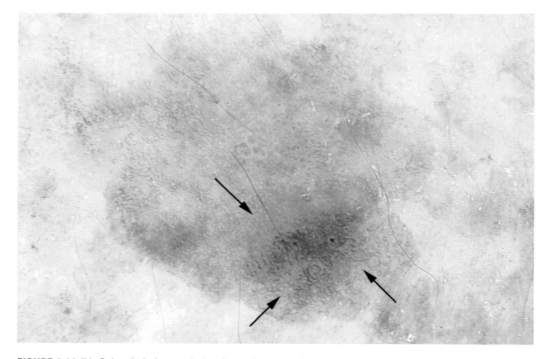

FIGURE 6.32 (b) Seborrheic keratosis (surface microscopy)
This lesion has areas of light brown fingerprint-like structures (such as delineated by arrows) which characterize some flat seborrheic keratoses (and some solar lentigo, from which they may arise). While the fingerprint-like structures are more curvilinear than pigment network structures seen in melanocytic lesions, sometimes it can be difficult to distinguish these from each other. Note also the areas of moth-eaten edge at the inferior margin of the lesion.

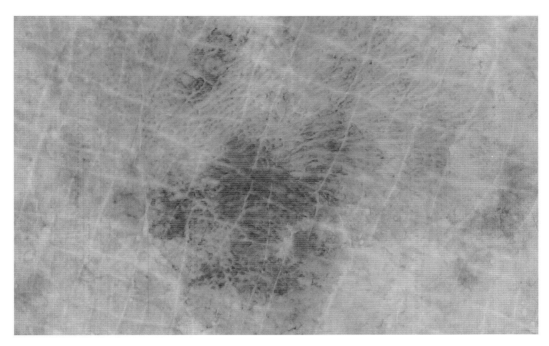

FIGURE 6.33 Seborrheic keratosis (dermoscopy)
Here another variant of ridges forming linear structures like fingerprint areas is seen throughout this flat seborrheic keratosis.

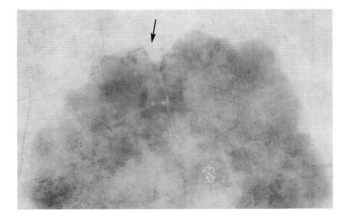

FIGURE 6.34 Seborrheic keratosis (dermoscopy)
In some flat seborrheic keratoses a uniform pigment background can be seen. Note also the moth eaten edge (arrow). There is a clear morphological overlap between solar lentigo and flat seborrheic keratoses both histologically and under dermoscopic examination.

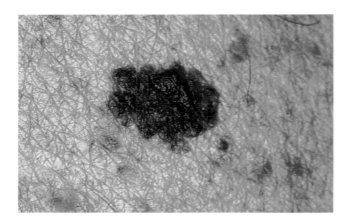

FIGURE 6.35 (a) Seborrheic keratosis (clinical view)

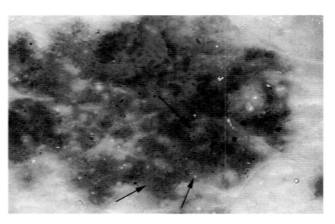

FIGURE 6.35 (b) Seborrheic keratosis (dermoscopy)

In an uncommon variant of seborrheic keratosis areas of well defined multiple blue-gray globules may be seen (arrows). In this lesion the absent true network and presence of multiple milia help to make the diagnosis.

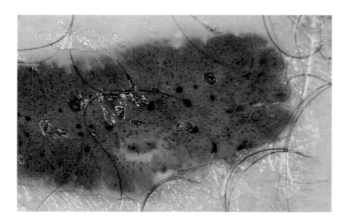

FIGURE 6.36 Seborrheic keratosis (dermoscopy)

In this lesion multiple blue-gray globules are seen throughout the lesion. Here, the additional presence of irregular crypts and lack of pigment network confirm the diagnosis.

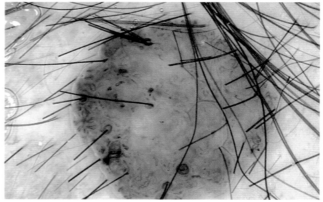

FIGURE 6.37 Seborrheic keratosis (dermoscopy)

Diffuse blue-gray pigmentation is seen in some pigmented seborrheic keratoses. This lesion also has a well-demarcated border, relatively regular distribution of hairpin loops of telangiectasia and scattered irregular crypts that all help to confirm the diagnosis. However, in some cases differentiating these from melanocytic lesions can be difficult.

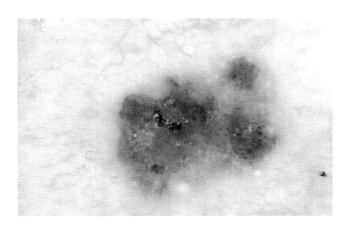

FIGURE 6.38 Seborrheic keratosis (dermoscopy)

In this atypical lesion the presence of multiple colors and areas resembling blue-white veil encourage the initial diagnosis of invasive melanoma. However the combination of a well demarcated border, multiple large milia-like cysts, absent network, and focus of multiple large, blue-gray globules confirm the diagnosis.

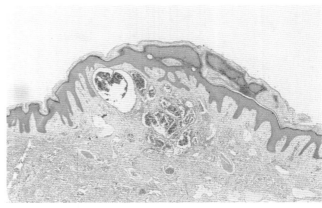

FIGURE 6.39 Hemangioma (histopathology)

This section shows a hemangioma composed of large dilated blood vessels (cavernous). Hemangiomas can also be composed of small vessels (capillary) or a mixture of both elements. Magnification ×10 (H & E stain).

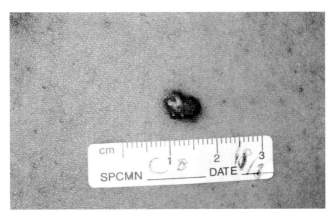

FIGURE 6.40 (a) Hemangioma (clinical view)

Clinically, hemangiomas can have elements of black pigmentation within the lesion. This may result in the inclusion of melanoma in the differential diagnosis.

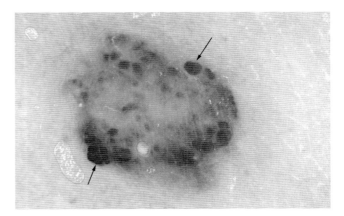

FIGURE 6.40 (b) Hemangioma (dermoscopy)

The hallmark of the hemangioma under dermoscopy is the presence of a red-blue color that in the majority of cases is the solitary color. In addition, the majority have ovoid, discrete red-blue areas (red-blue lacunes) as seen here (arrows). Note that the corresponding areas of black pigmentation seen clinically are red-blue under dermoscopy.

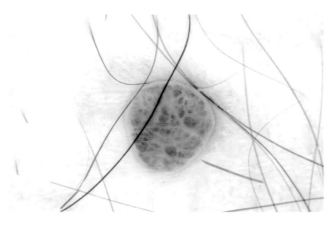

FIGURE 6.41 Hemangioma (dermoscopy)
Some hemangiomas have distinct scar-like depigmentation surrounding the vascular spaces.

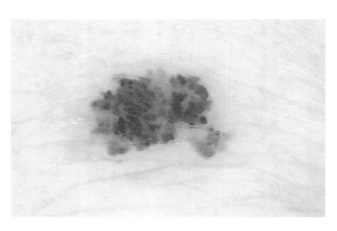

FIGURE 6.44 Hemangioma (dermoscopy)
Blue-white veil, a characteristic of invasive melanoma, can never be diagnosed in the presence of multiple red-blue lacunes.

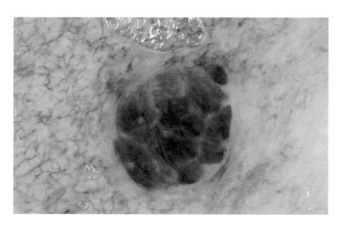

FIGURE 6.42 Hemangioma (dermoscopy)
The color of the red-blue areas varies in hemangiomas from predominantly red (Figure 6.41), a mixture of red and blue (as seen here), to, less commonly, almost purely blue (Figure 6.43).

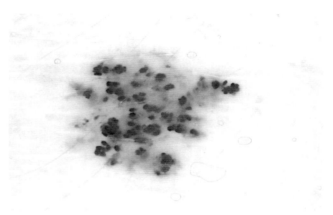

FIGURE 6.45 Hemangioma (dermoscopy)
Classic, multiple red-blue lacunes are seen in this hemangioma.

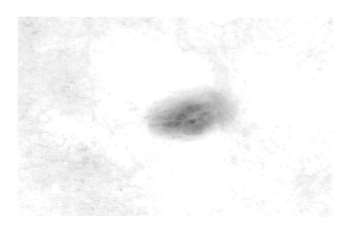

FIGURE 6.43 Hemangioma (dermoscopy)

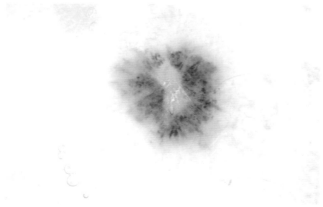

FIGURE 6.46 Hemangioma (dermoscopy)
Note the central area of scar-like depigmentation in this hemangioma. Fibrosis is a histopathological finding seen in some hemangiomas.

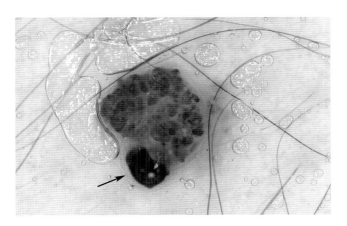

FIGURE 6.47 Hemangioma (dermoscopy)
When focal thrombi occur in hemangioma the lacunes are seen as dark red to black (arrow).

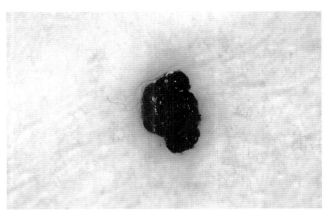

FIGURE 6.49 Cutaneous thrombus (dermoscopy)
Cutaneous thrombi often present as rapidly changing, ink-black plaques or papules, sometimes mimicking melanoma. However, the solitary dermoscopic finding of uniform black pigmentation, without any other feature, excludes the diagnosis of melanoma.

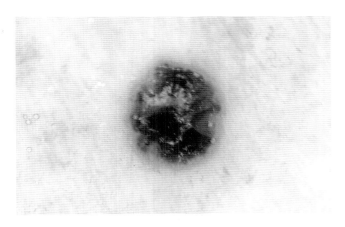

FIGURE 6.48 Hemangioma (dermoscopy)
Again vessels contaning fibrin thrombi result in the darker red areas seen. In addition, areas of scale and crust are seen. Such findings are common in angiokeratomas.

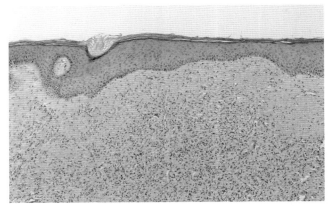

FIGURE 6.50 Dermatofibroma (histiocytoma) (histopathology)
This lesion shows a dermal collection of spindle-shaped cells which are fibroblastic cells. Histiocytes may also be present. Dermatofibromas are usually well circumscribed but not encapsulated. They may show overlying epidermal hyperplasia with increased basal pigmentation. Magnification ×25 (H & E stain).

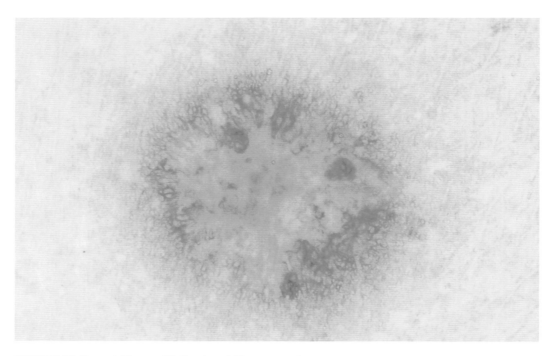

FIGURE 6.51 Dermatofibroma (histiocytoma) (dermoscopy)

The commonest pattern of the dermatofibroma is the central white scar-like patch with a peripheral delicate pigment network. This network is due to increased basal pigmentation in combination with epidermal thickening. While this lesion can be diagnosed with dermoscopy alone, dermoscopy usually only aids the characteristic clinical findings of a button-hard lesion with dimpling when pressed at the edges (pinch sign).

FIGURE 6.52 Dermatofibroma (histiocytoma) (dermoscopy)

Here a central white network is seen. This may be difficult to distinguish between the negative network seen in some melanocytic lesions.

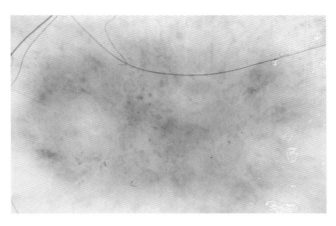

FIGURE 6.53 Dermatofibroma (histiocytoma) (dermoscopy)
Here the white scar-like patch is found in a multifocal distribution. Areas of erythema are also seen in some dermatofibroma. In addition, some dotted vessels are found centrally. Dotted vessels are the most common vessel type in dermatofibromas.

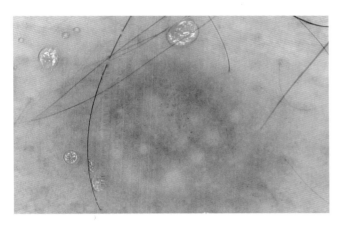

FIGURE 6.54 Dermatofibroma (histiocytoma) (dermoscopy)
Again the white scar-like patches are found in a multifocal distribution with surrounding homogeneous brown pigmentation. Ninety-four percent of dermatofibromas have combinations of the basic morphological structures of fine discrete network, white scar-like patch, white network, and homogenous brown or red-blue pigmentation.

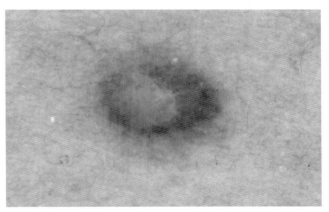

FIGURE 6.55 Dermatofibroma (histiocytoma) (dermoscopy)
This lesion has a central white scar-like patch with surrounding red-blue homogeneous pigmentation.

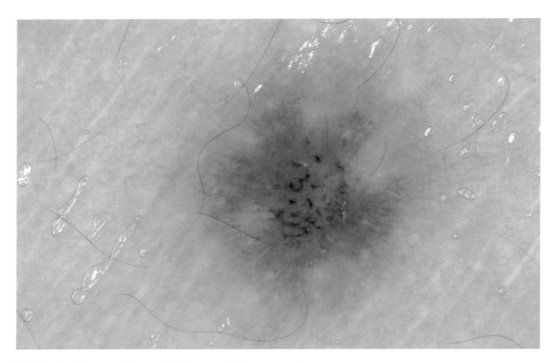

FIGURE 6.56 Dermatofibroma (histiocytoma) (dermoscopy)

This lesion has homogeneous red-brown pigmentation which merges with a delicate network at the periphery. Variable degrees of epidermal lichenification may cause crypts and fissure-like areas as seen centrally here. Also note areas of perifollicular depigmentation which may mimic multifocal scar-like patches.

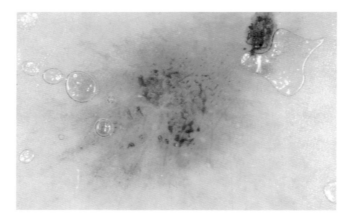

FIGURE 6.57 Dermatofibroma (histiocytoma) (dermoscopy)

The presence of fissures suggests the possible diagnosis of a seborrheic keratosis. However, clinically this was a hard lesion with a positive pinch test, confirming the diagnosis of a dermatofibroma. Note the subtle central white scar-like patch.

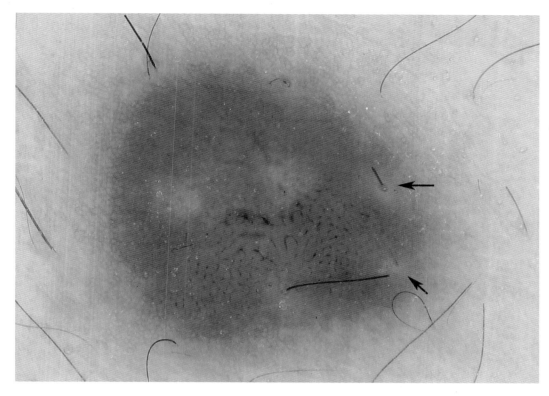

FIGURE 6.58 Dermatofibroma (histiocytoma) (dermoscopy)
This lesion has homogeneous red-blue pigmentation with areas of perifollicular depigmentation (arrows). The homogeneous pigmentation merges with a delicate peripheral pigment network. Centrally areas of brown globule-like structures are due to small crypts in the thickened epidermis.

FIGURE 6.59 (a) Epidermal nevus—Becker's nevus (clinical view)
Becker's nevi (pigmented hairy epidermal nevi) are first noted primarily in adolescent males.

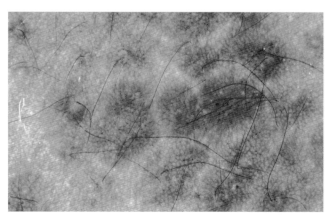

FIGURE 6.59 (b) Epidermal nevus—Becker's nevus (dermoscopy)
While this is not a melanocytic nevus, histopathologically the elongated rete ridges in combination with increased epidermal pigmentation lead to a prominence of the normal pigmented network of the skin (as seen here).

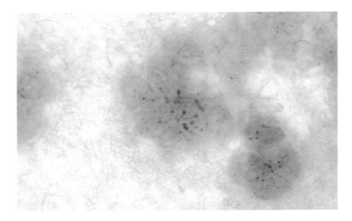

FIGURE 6.60 Epidermal nevus—verrucous (dermoscopy)
Verrucous epidermal nevi can occur at birth and usually during the first decade of life. They can be any shape, but many form elongated linear extensions. Under dermoscopy the absent pigment network confirms the non-melanocytic nature of the nevus. However, in this case the presence of multiple fissures and crypts makes any distinction between a verrucous epidermal nevus and a seborrheic keratosis possible only by the clinical history. (Seborrheic keratoses never occur in the first decade.)

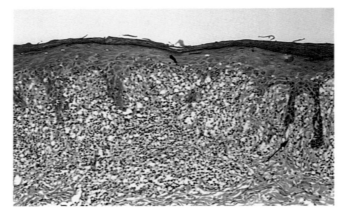

FIGURE 6.61 Lichen planus-like keratosis (histopathology)*
In this lichen planus-like keratosis there is a marked inflammatory infiltrate in the superficial dermis which also involves the dermo-epidermal junction (lichenoid reaction). Within the inflammatory infiltrate there are scattered macrophages containing melanin pigment (melanophages). Adjacent to the inflammatory infiltrate there are changes suggestive of a solar lentigo (arrow) with pigmented elongated rete ridges. Magnification ×25 (H & E stain).

* This photograph was kindly provided by Dr Graham Mason, Melbourne, Australia.

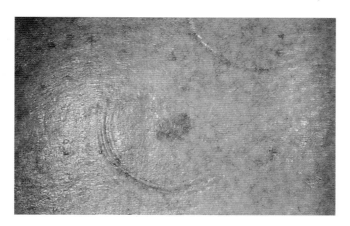

FIGURE 6.62 (a) Lichen planus-like keratosis (clinical view)[†]

Lichen planus-like keratoses are most commonly seen as single lesions on the upper extremities, face and chest. They usually have the history of a preceding pigmented macule/plaque (solar lentigo or seborrheic keratosis), are often rapidly changing, and many are pruritic (with a range of other abnormal sensations).

[†] *Photograph kindly provided by Dr Harold Rabinovitz, Miami, USA.*

FIGURE 6.62 (b) Lichen planus-like keratosis (dermoscopy)[‡]

A common presentation is an area of diffuse multiple blue-gray dots (melanophages) on a uniform tan background.

[‡] *Photograph kindly provided by Dr Harold Rabinovitz, Miami, USA.*

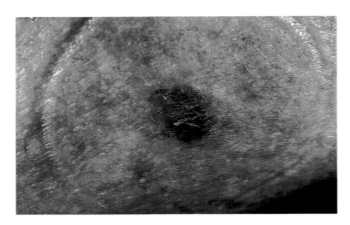

FIGURE 6.63 (a) Lichen planus-like keratosis (clinical view)[¶]
The color may vary from dark dusky violaceous or rust color to pink or crimson.

[¶] *Photograph kindly provided by Dr Harold Rabinovitz, Miami, USA.*

FIGURE 6.63 (b) Lichen planus-like keratosis (dermoscopy)**
Lichen planus-like keratoses are thought to be most often regressing solar lentigo or seborrheic keratoses. Here, localized multiple blue-gray dots are seen within a lesion of uniform tan background, areas of fine pigment network and borderline fingerprint-like structures (i.e. regressing solar lentigo). In some lesions, where a more distinct network is seen, biopsy is indicated to exclude regressing melanoma.

** *Photograph kindly provided by Dr Harold Rabinovitz, Miami, USA.*

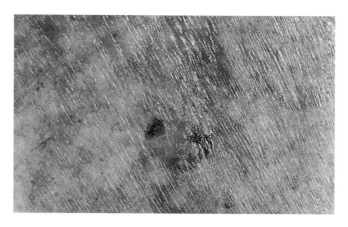

FIGURE 6.64 (a) Lichen planus-like keratosis (clinical view)[††]

[††] *Photograph kindly provided by Dr Harold Rabinovitz, Miami, USA.*

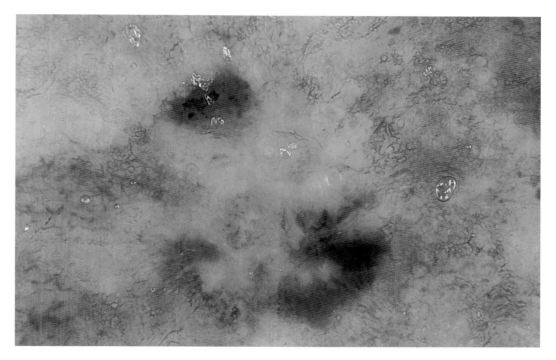

FIGURE 6.64 (b) Lichen planus-like keratosis (dermoscopy)[‡‡]
Here areas of regression (localized multiple blue-gray dots and depigmentation) are seen with areas of seborrheic keratosis (distinct brown pigmentation, irregular crypts and absent network). However, a confident exclusion of regressing melanoma cannot be made and biopsy was necessary to confirm the diagnosis (see also Figure 2.61).

[‡‡] *Photograph kindly provided by Dr Harold Rabinovitz, Miami, USA.*

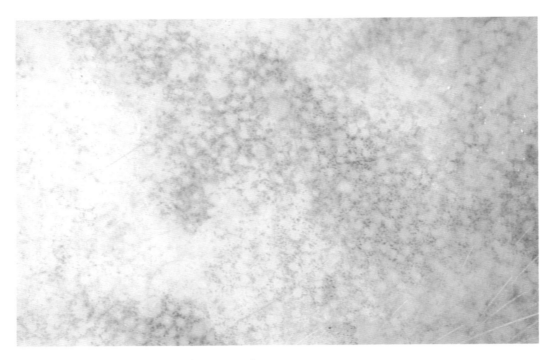

FIGURE 6.65 Pigment incontinence (dermoscopy)

The solitary presence of multiple blue-gray dots (dermal melanophages, i.e. melanin-containing macrophages) occurs from melanin being shed from the epidermis. Pigment incontinence can occur in a variety of non-melanocytic-derived pathologies and is often found following inflammation or destruction of the basal layer of the epidermis (e.g. lichenoid eruptions). In the lesion shown, the melanophages are high in the dermis and appear gray-brown in color (rather than their more classical blue-gray color).

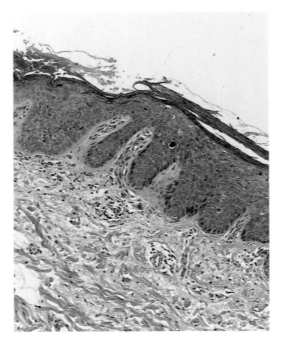

FIGURE 6.66 Bowen's disease (in situ squamous cell carcinoma) (histopathology)

The epidermis shows full thickness atypia and surface scale. In this example there is prominent basal pigmentation. Small blood vessels are present in the dermis. Magnification ×50 (H & E stain).

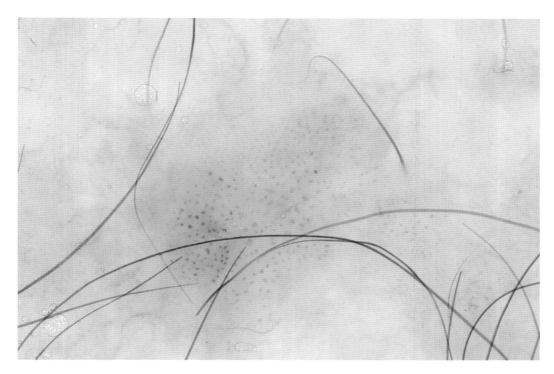

FIGURE 6.67 (a) Bowen's disease (in situ squamous cell carcinoma) (dermoscopy)
Bowen's disease usually presents as erythematous plaques on chronic sun exposed sites. Under dermoscopy they have characteristic glomerular vessels in combination with scale.

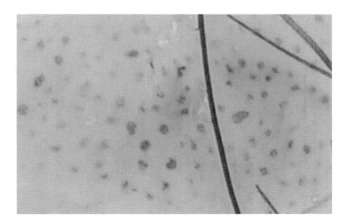

FIGURE 6.67 (b) Bowen's disease (in situ squamous cell carcinoma) (dermoscopy: magnified view)
The glomerular vessels are easily seen with normal ×10 magnified hand-held surface microscopes.

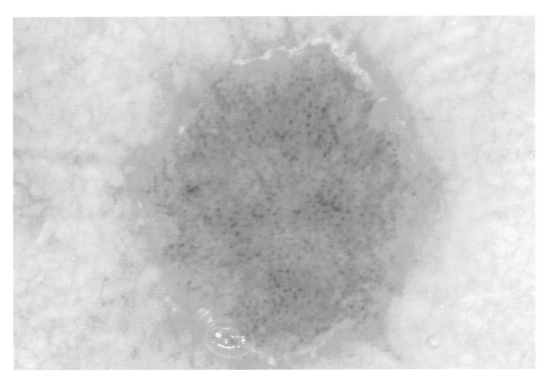

FIGURE 6.68 Psoriasis (dermoscopy)
The dermoscopic features of plaque psoriasis overlap substantially with non-pigmented Bowen's disease, with psoriatic plaques tending to have a more regular distribution of vessels compared with Bowen's. However, the multiple nature and distribution of psoriatic plaques usually enables easy distinction between the two entities.

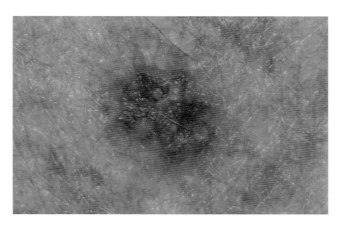

FIGURE 6.69 (a) Pigmented Bowen's disease (in situ squamous cell carcinoma) (clinical)[§§]

In anglo-celtic races pigmented Bowen's disease is less common. However, rarely Bowen's disease can present as pigmented scaly plaques.

[§§] *This photograph was kindly provided by Dr Alan Cameron, Australia.*

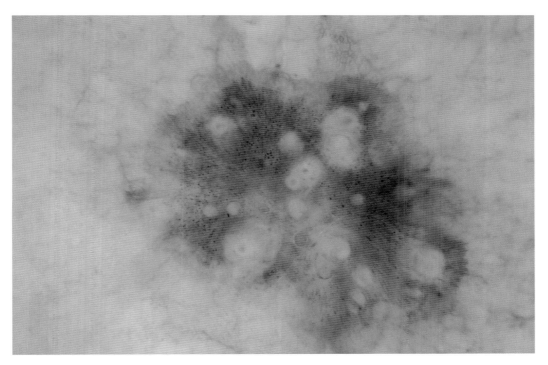

FIGURE 6.69 (b) Pigmented Bowen's disease (in situ squamous cell carcinoma) (dermoscopy)[¶¶]

When pigmented, Bowen's disease may have brown globules under dermoscopy mimicking a melanocytic lesion.

[¶¶] *This photograph was kindly provided by Dr Alan Cameron, Australia.*

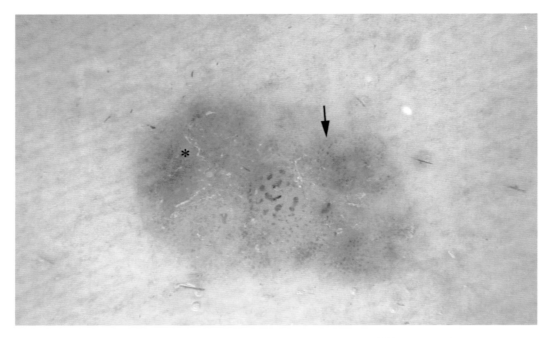

FIGURE 6.70 Pigmented Bowen's disease (in situ squamous cell carcinoma) (dermoscopy)***
Here homogeneous brown pigmentation (asterisk), scale, brown globules (arrow) and distinct central glomerular vessels are seen.

*** This photograph was kindly provided by Dr Giuseppe Argenziano, Napoli, Italy.

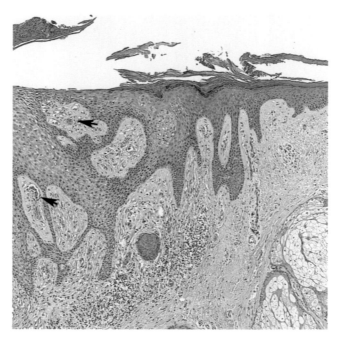

FIGURE 6.71 Clear cell acanthoma (histopathology)
Clear cell acanthoma is seen on the left and exhibits thickened epidermis composed of clear cells and is sharply demarcated from the normal epidermis on the right. Note the dilated vessels in the dermis (arrows). Magnification ×25 (H & E stain).

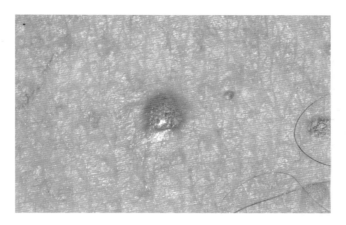

FIGURE 6.72 (a) Clear cell acanthoma (clinical)[†††]

Clear cell acanthoma are benign lesions that usually present as solitary, slowly growing pink, or red dome-shaped nodules, and are most commonly found on the lower legs of middle-aged or elderly people.

[†††] *This photograph was kindly provided by Dr Giuseppi Argenziano, Napoli, Italy.*

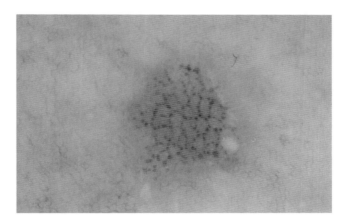

FIGURE 6.72 (b) Clear cell acanthoma (dermoscopy)[‡‡‡]

These lesions are particularly striking under dermoscopy with the characteristic enlarged dotted/glomerular vessels in a reticular/linear or so-called "string of pearls" pattern.

[‡‡‡] *This photograph was kindly provided by Dr Giuseppi Argenziano, Napoli, Italy.*

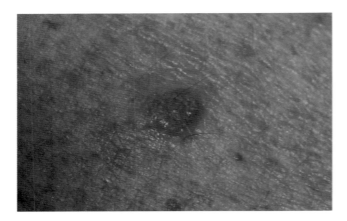

FIGURE 6.73 (a) Clear cell acanthoma (clinical)§§§

§§§ *This photograph was kindly provided by Dr Giuseppi Argenziano, Napoli, Italy.*

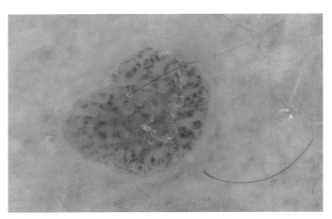

FIGURE 6.73 (b) Clear cell acanthoma (dermoscopy)¶¶¶

Again the glomerular vessels are found in a reticular/linear string of pearls pattern.

¶¶¶ *This photograph was kindly provided by Dr Giuseppi Argenziano, Napoli, Italy.*

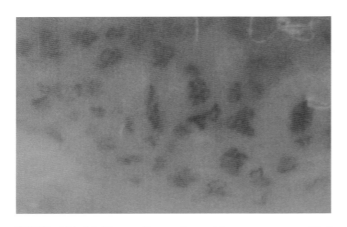

FIGURE 6.73 (c) Clear cell acanthoma (dermoscopy: magnified view)****

The individual glomerular vessels are difficult to distinguish between Bowen's, plaque psoriasis, and clear cell acanthoma. However, the overall pattern of the vessels contrasts clear cell acanthoma from the former two lesions.

**** *This photograph was kindly provided by Dr Giuseppi Argenziano, Napoli, Italy*

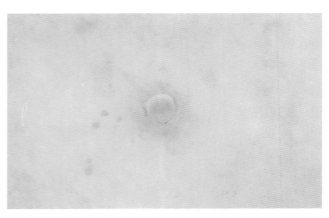

FIGURE 6.74 Rapidly appearing blue nodule (dermoscopy)

This patient presented with a sudden appearance of a small blue nodule. The surface microscopic findings are of a well-demarcated oval body with two lateral brown extensions. Diagnosis—a burrowing tick. The application of immersion oil facilitated the diagnosis and successfully treated the condition at the same time.

CHAPTER SEVEN

TWO-STEP PROCEDURE FOR DIAGNOSIS OF PIGMENTED SKIN LESIONS

A simplified dermoscopy method for the diagnosis of pigmented skin lesions has been developed.[1,2] The "first step" involves identifying the lesion as either melanocytic in origin (ephelis, lentigo, all nevi, melanoma) or non-melanocytic (seborrheic keratosis, BCC, hemangioma, dermatofibroma). Although the ephelis and solar lentigo are not strictly melanocytic-derived lesions, they are included as such in the first step. If the lesion is identified as melanocytic, a "second step" procedure differentiates benign melanocytic lesions from melanoma.

While a number of second step procedures have been published (see the introduction to Chapter 5), we describe only one here. It is important to understand that the two-step procedure is not suitable for the diagnosis of amelanotic/hypomelanotic melanoma since these lesions often fail in both the first and second steps (see Chapter 5). The following two-step procedure is used to describe the "unknowns", as accessed on www.mhhe.com/au/dermoscopyatlas3e.

First Step

Diagnostic algorithm for differentiating melanocytic from non-melanocytic lesions

Modified according to Kreusch, Stolz, and Menzies.

Criteria for a melanocytic lesion

- Pigment network—pseudo-network (see exception 1)
- Aggregated brown or black globules (including variant of cobblestone pattern)
- Pseudopods or radial streaming (circumferential or focally present)
- Homogeneous blue pigmentation (see exception 2)
- Parallel pattern (on palms/soles)

Criteria for seborrheic keratosis

- Multiple milia-like cysts (see exception 3)
- Irregular crypts (see exception 3)
- Fissures/ridges
- Light-brown fingerprint-like structures (see exception 5)

Criteria for pigmented basal cell carcinoma

Absent pigment network and one or more of:
- arborizing vessels
- leaf-like areas
- large blue-gray ovoid nests
- multiple blue-gray globules (see exception 4)
- spoke wheel areas
- ulceration

Criteria for vascular lesion

- Widespread red-blue lacunes
- Red-bluish to red-black homogeneous areas

If none of the listed criteria diagnose as melanocytic

Exception 1 A delicate, annular pigment network is commonly seen also in dermatofibroma (clue for diagnosis of dermatofibroma: central white scar-like patch or white network). Network structures are sometimes seen in seborrheic keratoses.

Exception 2 Homogeneous blue pigmentation (hallmark of blue nevus) is also seen (uncommonly) in some hemangiomas and BCCs.

Exception 3 Multiple milia-like cysts and crypts can occur in occasional dermal or congenital nevi.

Exception 4 In some rare cases of seborrheic keratoses multiple blue-gray globules can be seen. Usually other features of seborrheic keratoses in these lesions help to make the diagnosis.

Exception 5 In solar lentigo (from which some seborrheic keratoses arise), and more rarely in lentigo maligna, light-brown fingerprint-like structures can be seen. In both of these situations, areas of pigment network (true or pseudo-network) are usually also found. If only light-brown fingerprint-like structures are seen without other features of seborrheic keratoses, such lesions should be considered as melanocytic in origin and the second step performed.

Second Step (used if first step diagnosis is melanocytic)

Diagnostic algorithm for differentiating benign melanocytic lesions from melanoma

Method for diagnosis of invasive and in situ (non-lentigo maligna melanoma)[3]

Negative Features (both cannot be found)

- Symmetrical pigmentation pattern
- Presence of only a single color

Positive Features (at least one feature found)

- Blue-white veil
- Multiple brown dots
- Pseudopods
- Radial streaming
- Scar-like depigmentation
- Peripheral black dots/globules
- Multiple (5–6) colors
- Multiple blue-gray dots (*see* exception 6)
- Broadened network

Additional positive features for diagnosis of lentigo maligna[4]

- Rhomboidal structures
- Annular granular pattern

- Asymmetric pigmented follicular openings
- Slate gray dots/globules

Additional positive features for diagnosis of melanoma on palms/soles[5,6]

- Parallel ridge pattern (flat component)
- Irregular diffuse pigmentation with variable shades from tan to black
- >7 mm diameter without typical parallel furrow/lattice or uniform fibrillar/filamentous patterns

Exception 6 Melanocytic nevi may have multiple blue-gray dots occupying less than 10% of the lesion without other positive features of melanoma. A diagnosis of lichen planus-like keratosis can be made when only features of seborrheic keratoses in addition to multiple blue-gray dots are found.

References

1. Soyer, H, Argenziano, G, Chimenti, S, Menzies, S, Pehamberger, H, Rabinovitz, H, Stolz, W, Kopf, A. *Dermoscopy of Pigmented Skin Lesions.* Milan, Italy: Edra: 2001.

2. Argenziano, G, Soyer, HP, Chimenti, S, et al. Dermoscopy of pigmented skin lesions: results of a consensus meeting via the internet. *J Am Acad Dermatol* 2003; 48: 679–93.

3. Menzies, S, Ingvar, C, Crotty, K, McCarthy, W. Frequency and morphologic characteristics of invasive melanomas lacking specific surface microscopic features. *Arch Dermatol* 1996; 132: 1178–82.

4. Schiffner, R, Schiffner-Rohe, J, Vogt, T, Landthaler, M, Wlotzke, U, Cognetta, A, Stolz, W. Improvement of early recognition of lentigo maligna using dermatoscopy. *J Am Acad Dermatol* 2000; 42: 25–32.

5. Saida, T, Miyazaki, A, Oguchi, S, Ishihara, Y, et al. Significance of dermoscopic patterns in detecting malignant melanoma on acral volar skin: results of a multicenter study in Japan. *Arch Dermatol* 2004; 140: 1233–8.

6. Saida, T, Koga, H. Dermoscopic patterns of acral melanocytic nevi: their variations, changes, and significance. *Arch Dermatol* 2007; 143: 1423–6.

CHAPTER EIGHT

COMPUTERIZED (DIGITAL) MONITORING OF MELANOCYTIC LESIONS

Digital (computerized) dermoscopy systems have undergone widespread investigation in recent times. These systems can be divided into three categories. First are those used to store images for viewing by clinicians in a conventional or telemedicine setting.[1-8] Second are those used in combination with image analysis that aim for automated diagnosis.[9,10] Third are those used for the monitoring of lesions for morphological change.[11-25] Digital dermoscopy monitoring of melanocytic lesions can be found in two settings: long-term surveillance over a 6- to 12-month period[11-14,16-24] or short-term surveillance over 3 months.[15,16,19,21,25] Currently, little is known about the natural history of monitoring non-melanocytic lesions. However, lesions such as seborrheic keratoses and lichen planus-like keratoses are known to change rapidly and therefore should not be monitored. For these reasons the following refers to the monitoring of exclusively melanocytic-derived lesions (ephelis, lentigo, nevi, and melanoma).

The advantage of sequential dermoscopy digital monitoring is that a *significant proportion of melanomas detected using the technique lack specific dermoscopy features of melanoma.*[15-19,25] Indeed, approximately two-thirds of melanomas detected using short-term monitoring and one-third using long-term monitoring are dermoscopically featureless.[16] Finally, when applied correctly, the technique is safe. In the two largest series describing melanomas detected using digital monitoring, the median Breslow thickness was in situ melanoma and all invasive melanoma were less than 0.9 mm thick.[16,25]

Long-term (12 month) monitoring

Here, images are stored from lesions that are confidently diagnosed as non-melanoma, and can be used to detect early melanoma at standard follow-up surveillance periods. The largest early study[14] defined the following "significant" changes that required excision of the lesion over a median 12 month monitoring period (50% followed up from 8–20 months):

- enlargement or shape change
- regression
- change in color (appearance of new colors)
- appearance of known melanoma dermoscopic features

Such changes occur in approximately 4–5% of monitored melanocytic nevi.[14,17,18] Of these significantly changed lesions, 12% are early melanoma.[14] Within such significantly changed lesions, nevi tend to enlarge symmetrically over time, whereas melanoma tends to enlarge asymmetrically. Furthermore, over the long-term monitoring period, observation of broadening of the network, increased black dots/globules, and focal increase in pigmentation are more predictive of changes in melanoma versus nevi.[16] The "non-significant" changes found in 28% of monitored lesions are a darker or lighter appearance, changes in the number or distribution of brown globules, decrease in the number of black dots, disappearance of an inflammatory reaction or disappearance of parts of the pigment network and replacement by diffuse light brown pigmentation. Such changes do not require excision biopsy.

Both atypical and banal nevi change in size over long-term monitoring more frequently in young people. Thirteen percent of banal nevi show size increase in people 0–20 years of age, whereas only 1.5% enlarge in adults older than 40 years.[13] Similarly 10% of atypical nevi enlarge in people younger than 28 years of age in contrast to only 3% in adults older than 48 years.[20] Finally, symmetrical nevi with multiple peripheral brown globules can rapidly increase in size and therefore should not be monitored.

Short-term (3 month) monitoring

In contrast to long-term monitoring of "baseline" images over a standard surveillance period, suspicious melanocytic lesions with moderate atypia that do not meet the dermoscopy criteria for melanoma, or lesions that have some minor atypia with a recent patient history of change, can undergo short-term computerized monitoring. In the case of moderately atypical nevi, these lesions should be flat or only superficially raised. This is to avoid monitoring an advanced melanoma. The criteria for excising lesions over a 3-month period[15] (range 2.5–4.5 months) are:

ANY change except:

- increase or decrease in milia-like cysts
- diffuse decrease or increase in pigmentation without architectural change (solar change)
- increase in size of Spitz nevi or nevi with multiple peripheral brown globules

In the case of solar change, diffuse pigmentation change of the normal surrounding skin (tanning or lightening of the skin) usually parallels the changes seen within the lesion. It should also be noted that sun exposure can induce increased irregularity in nevi over the short-term monitoring period.[26] To avoid incorrect interpretation of monitored changes, patients should avoid direct sun exposure of their monitored nevi.

In the largest series of short-term monitoring, 84% of benign melanocytic lesions do not change over a 2.5–4.5 month period (median 3 months).[25] Of the changed lesions, 12% are early melanoma.[15] These lesions usually show none of the classic dermoscopic features of melanoma and can only be identified by change following computerized monitoring. Unlike in long-term monitoring no specific type of change predicts whether a lesion will be melanoma or benign under short-term monitoring.[16] Importantly, 99.2% of lesions remaining unchanged at 2.5–4.5 months are benign.[25] While 94% of melanoma (non-lentigo maligna type) will change during the short-term interval, only 75% of lentigo maligna change at this time interval. For this reason, a second monitored interval between 6–12 months following the baseline image is recommended where the diagnosis of lentigo maligna is being excluded. Finally, a patient history of change in a lesion does not influence the outcome of monitoring or final diagnosis of melanoma, i.e. if the patient reported a change there is no increased chance of subsequent change or melanoma diagnosis compared to patients who gave no history of change when taking their baseline (first) image.

References

1. Kenet, R, Kang, S, Kenet, B, et al. Clinical diagnosis of pigmented lesions using digital epiluminescence microscopy: grading protocol and atlas. *Arch Dermatol* 1993; 129: 157–74.

2. Piccolo, D, Smolle, J, Argenziano, G, et al. Teledermoscopy—results of a multicentre study on 43 pigmented skin lesions. *J Telemed Telecare* 2000; 6: 132–7.

3. Stanganelli, I, Serafini, M, Bucchi, L. A Cancer-registry-assisted evaluation of the accuracy of digital epiluminescence microscopy associated with clinical examination of pigmented skin lesions. *Dermatology* 2000; 200: 11–16.

4. Piccolo, D, Smolle J, Wolf, I, et al. Face-to-face diagnosis vs telediagnosis of pigmented skin tumors. *Arch Dermatol* 1999; 135: 1467–71.

5. Kittler, H, Seltenheim, M, Pehamberger, H, et al. Diagnostic informativeness of compressed digital epiluminescence microscopy images of pigmented skin lesions compared with photographs. *Melanoma Res* 1998; 8: 255–60.

6. Di Stefani, A, Zalaudek, I, Argenziano, G, Chimenti, S, Soyer, HP. Feasibility of a two-step teledermatologic approach for the management of patients with multiple pigmented skin lesions. *Dermatol Surg* 2007; 33: 686–92.

7. Bowns, IR, Collins, K, Walters, SJ, McDonagh, AJ. Telemedicine in dermatology: a randomised controlled trial. *Health Technol Assess* 2006; 10: iii–iv, ix–xi, 1–39.

8. Moreno-Ramirez, D, Ferrandiz, L, Galdeano, R, Camacho, FM. Teledermatoscopy as a triage system for pigmented lesions: a pilot study. *Clin Exp Dermatol* 2006; 31: 13–18.

9. Menzies, S W. Automated epiluminescence microscopy: Human vs machine in the diagnosis of melanoma. *Arch Dermatol* 1999; 135: 1538–40.

10. Vestergaard, ME, Menzies, SW. Automated diagnostic instruments for cutaneous melanoma. *Semin Cutan Med Surg* 2008; 27: 32–6.

11. Stolz, W, Schiffner, R, Pillet, L, et al. Improvement of monitoring of melanocytic skin lesions with the use of a computerized acquisition and surveillance unit with

a skin surface microscopic television camera. *J Am Acad Dermatol* 1996; 35: 202–7.

12. Braun, R, Lemonnier E, Guillod, J, et al. Two types of pattern modification detected on the follow-up of benign melanocytic skin lesions by digitized epiluminescence microscopy. *Melanoma Res* 1998; 8: 431–7.

13. Kittler, H, Seltenheim, M, Dawid, M, et al. Frequency and characteristics of enlarging common melanocytic nevi. *Arch Dermatol* 2000; 136: 316–20.

14. Kittler, H, Pehamberger, H, Wolff, K, et al. Follow-up of melanocytic skin lesions with digital epiluminescence microscopy: Patterns of modifications observed in early melanoma, atypical nevi, and common nevi. *J Am Acad Dermatol* 2000; 43: 467–76.

15. Menzies, S, Gutenev, A, Avramidis, M, Batrac, A, McCarthy, W. Short-term digital surface microscopy monitoring of atypical or changing melanocytic lesions. *Arch Dermatol* 2001; 137: 1583–9.

16. Kittler, H, Guitera, P, Riedl, E, Avramidis, M, Teban, L, Fiebiger, M, Weger, RA, Dawid, M, Menzies, SW. Identification of clinically featureless incipient melanoma using sequential dermoscopy imaging. *Arch Dermatol* 2006; 142: 1113–19.

17. Haenssle, HA, Krueger, U, Vente, C, et al. Results from an observational trial: digital epiluminescence microscopy follow-up of atypical nevi increases the sensitivity and the chance of success of conventional dermoscopy in detecting melanoma. *J Invest Dermatol* 2006; 126: 980–5.

18. Robinson, JK, Nickoloff, BJ. Digital epiluminescence microscopy monitoring of high-risk patients. *Arch Dermatol* 2004; 140: 49–56.

19. Skvara, H, Teban, L, Fiebiger, M, Binder, M, Kittler, H. Limitations of dermoscopy in the recognition of melanoma. *Arch Dermatol* 2005; 141: 155–60.

20. Bauer, J, Blum, A, Strohhacker, U, Garbe, C. Surveillance of patients at high risk for cutaneous malignant melanoma using digital dermoscopy. *Br J Dermatol* 2005; 152: 87–92.

21. Malvehy, J, Puig, S. Follow-up of melanocytic skin lesions with digital total-body photography and digital dermoscopy: a two-step method. *Clin Dermatol* 2002; 20: 297–304.

22. Schiffner, R, Schiffner-Rohe, J, Landthaler, M, Stolz, W. Long-term dermoscopic follow-up of melanocytic naevi: clinical outcome and patient compliance. *Br J Dermatol* 2003; 149: 79–86.

23. Fuller, SR, Bowen, GM, Tanner, B, Florell, SR, Grossman, D. Digital dermoscopic monitoring of atypical nevi in patients at risk for melanoma. *Dermatol Surg* 2007; 33: 1198–206.

24. Altamura, D, Zalaudek, I, Sera, F, Argenziano, G, Fargnoli, MC, Rossiello, L, Peris, K. Dermoscopic changes in acral melanocytic nevi during digital follow-up. *Arch Dermatol* 2007; 143: 1372–6.

25. Altamura, D, Avramidis, M, Menzies, SW. Assessment of the optimal interval for and sensitivity of short-term sequential digital dermoscopy monitoring for the diagnosis of melanoma. *Arch Dermatol* 2008; 144: 502–6.

26. Hofmann-Wellenhof, R, Wolf, P, Smolle, J, et al. Influence of UVB therapy on dermoscopic features of acquired melanocytic nevi. *J Am Acad Dermatol* 1997; 37: 559–63.

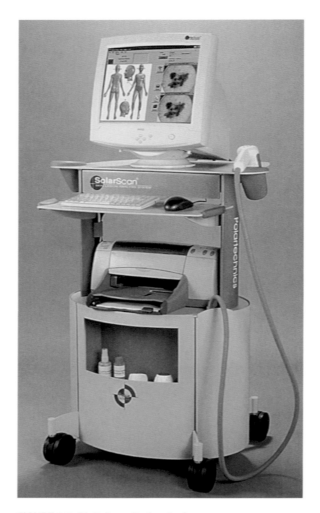

FIGURE 8.1 Digital monitoring devices

Currently, the most common method to monitor dermoscopy images of melanocytic lesions involves digital dermoscopy mega-pixel cameras or video instruments. Such instruments vary in their resolution, field of view and color calibration capability. The instrument shown here is the SolarScan (Polartechnics Ltd, Sydney). The following images have been taken using this instrument.

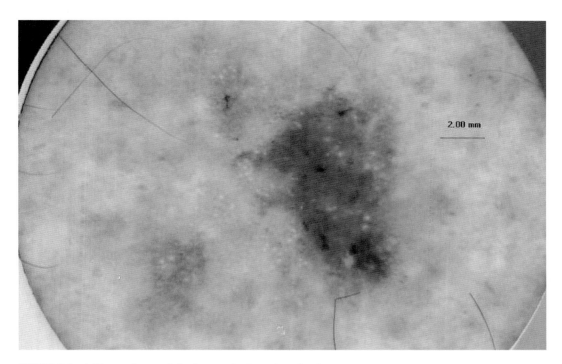

FIGURE 8.2 (a) Non-melanocytic lesion monitoring—baseline image
The 2 mm measurement bar shows the magnification seen in all the following images.

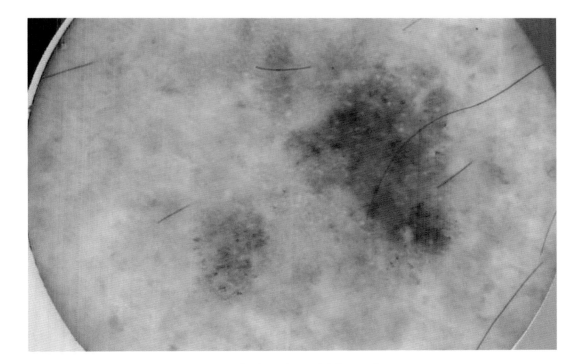

FIGURE 8.2 (b) Non-melanocytic lesion monitoring—3 month follow-up image
Currently, little is known about the natural history of monitoring non-melanocytic lesions. However, lesions such as seborrheic keratoses (as shown here) are known to change rapidly and therefore should not be monitored. For these reasons the following refers to the monitoring of exclusively melanocytic-derived lesions (ephelis, lentigo, nevi and melanoma).

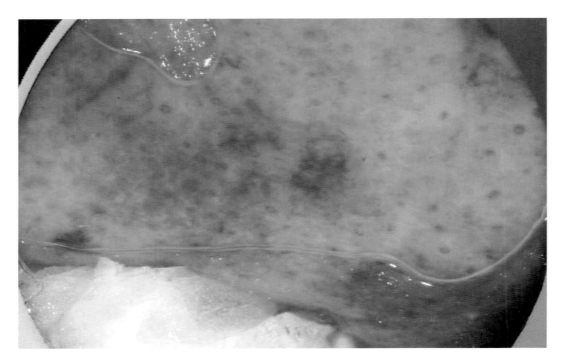

FIGURE 8.3 (a) Long-term monitoring—baseline image
In long-term surveillance images are stored from lesions that are more confidently diagnosed as non-melanoma, and can be used to detect early melanoma at standard follow-up surveillance periods (e.g. 6–12 months).

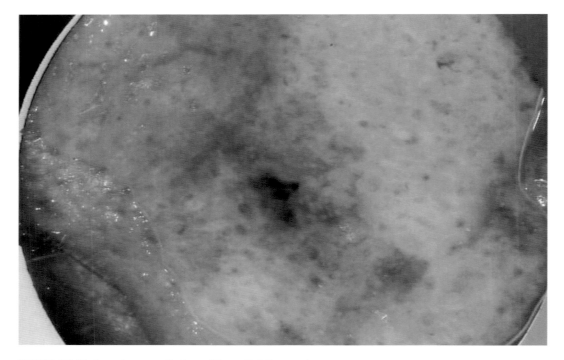

FIGURE 8.3 (b) Long-term monitoring—24 month follow-up image
Certain "significant" changes define the need to excise a lesion following long-term monitoring. The changes are enlargement or shape change, regression, change in color (appearance of new colors), or appearance of known melanoma dermoscopic features. Here, this nasal lesion has shown gross size, shape and color change over the 2-year monitoring period. Diagnosis: Lentigo maligna.

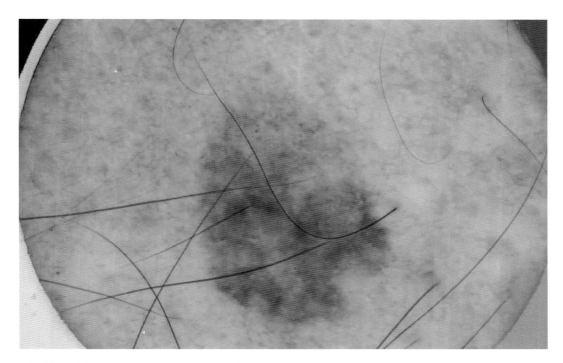

FIGURE 8.4 (a) Long-term monitoring—baseline image

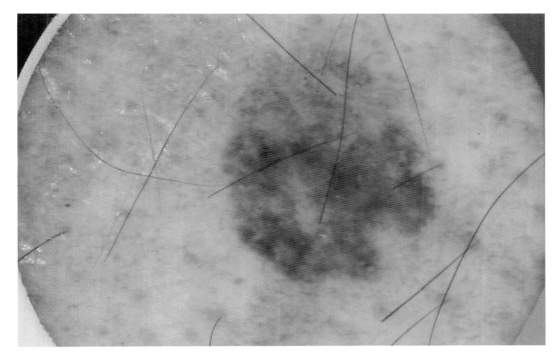

FIGURE 8.4 (b) Long-term monitoring—14 month follow-up image
This lesion has significantly increased in size over the monitoring period. Four percent of melanocytic lesions develop such "significant changes". However, only 12% of these lesions are found to be melanoma. When they enlarge over the long-term monitoring interval, 75% of nevi tend to increase in size symmetrically (as seen here) in contrast to melanoma which tends to increase asymmetrically. Diagnosis: Dysplastic compound nevus.

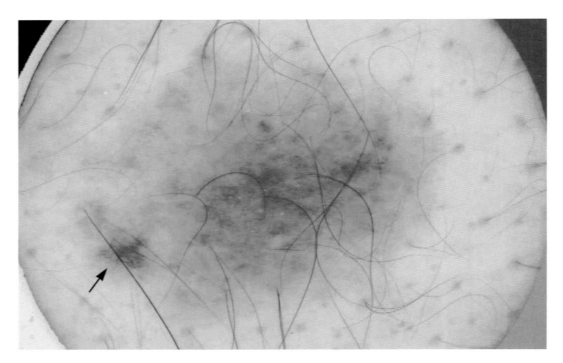

FIGURE 8.5 (a) Long-term monitoring—baseline image

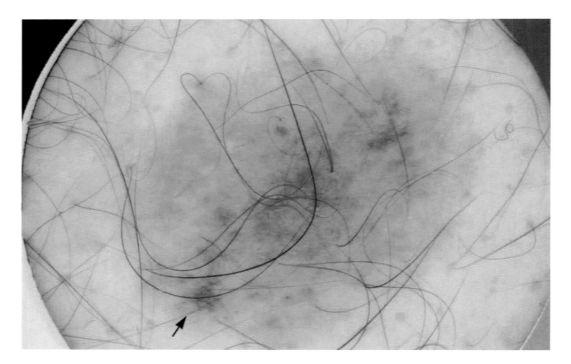

FIGURE 8.5 (b) Long-term monitoring—16 month follow-up image

The "non-significant" changes found in 28% of monitored lesions include disappearance of parts of the pigment network and replacement by a diffuse light brown pigmentation (as shown with arrow) and changes in the number or distribution of brown globules (as seen more subtly here). Other "non-significant" changes (not seen here) are a darker or lighter appearance, decrease in the number of black dots and disappearance of an inflammatory reaction. Such changes do not require excision biopsy. In addition, nevi with multiple peripheral brown globules (Figure 2.54) can rapidly increase in size and should not be monitored.

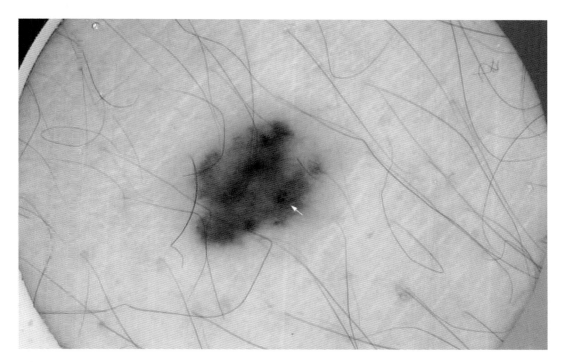

FIGURE 8.6 (a) Long-term monitoring—baseline image

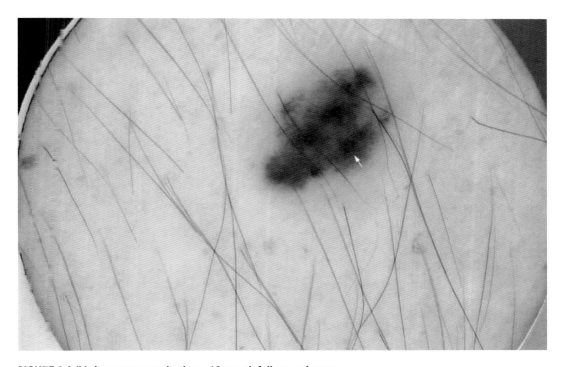

FIGURE 8.6 (b) Long-term monitoring—13 month follow-up image
This lesion has the "non-significant" change of loss of black dots/globules (arrow). No excision is warranted.

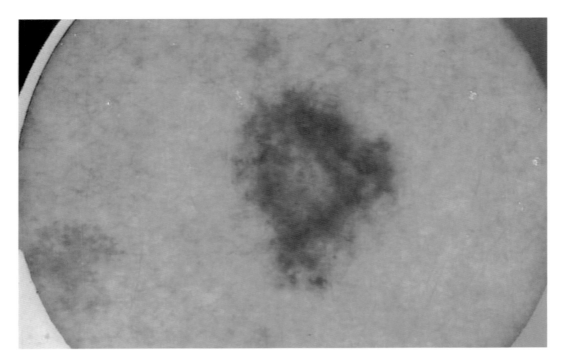

FIGURE 8.7 (a) Long-term monitoring—baseline image

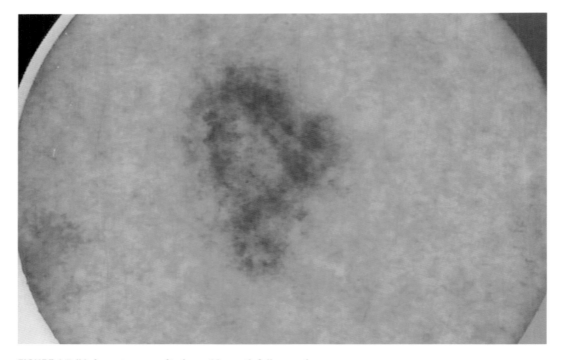

FIGURE 8.7 (b) Long-term monitoring—13 month follow-up image
This lesion has the "non-significant" changes of disappearance of an inflammatory reaction and change in distribution of brown globules. No excision is warranted.

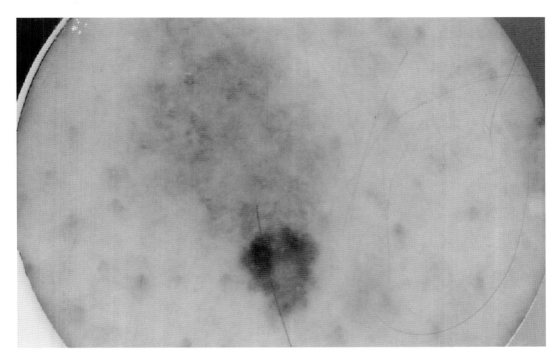

FIGURE 8.8 (a) **Long-term monitoring—baseline image**

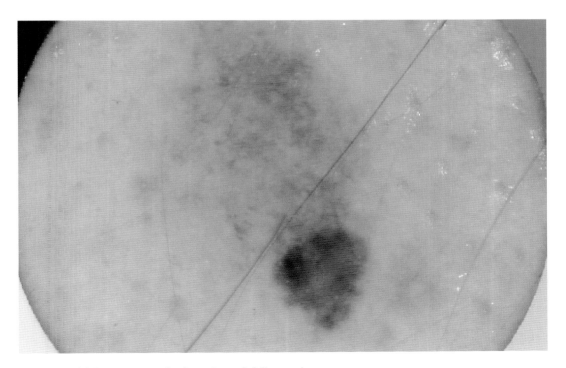

FIGURE 8.8 (b) **Long-term monitoring—9 month follow-up image**

Three changes in long-term monitored lesions are predictive of melanoma: observation of broadening of the network over time, increase in the number of black dots/globules, and as seen in this lesion a focal increase in pigmentation (in this case causing asymmetric enlargement of the lesion). Diagnosis: In situ melanoma.

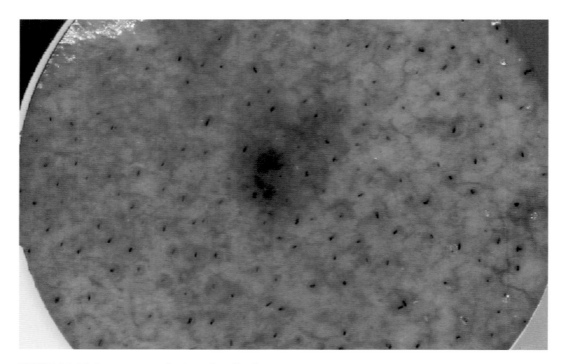

FIGURE 8.9 (a) Long-term monitoring—baseline image

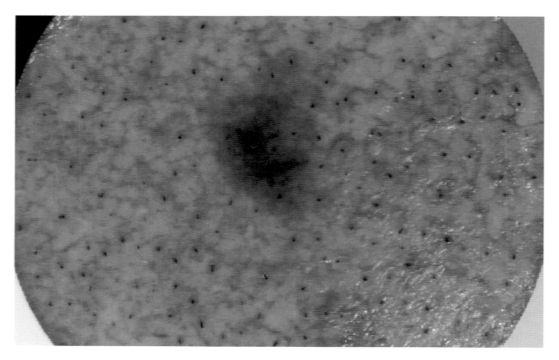

FIGURE 8.9 (b) Long-term monitoring—12 month follow-up image
Here both broadening of the network and focal increase in pigmentation is seen. Diagnosis: In situ melanoma.

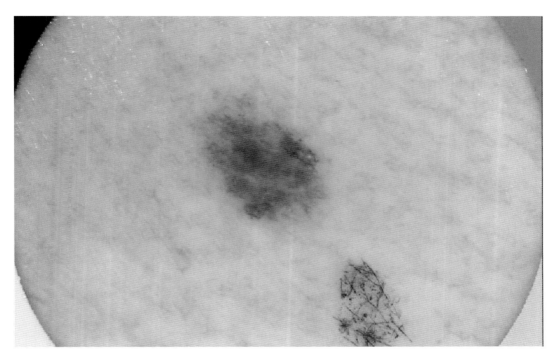

FIGURE 8.10 (a) Long-term monitoring—baseline image

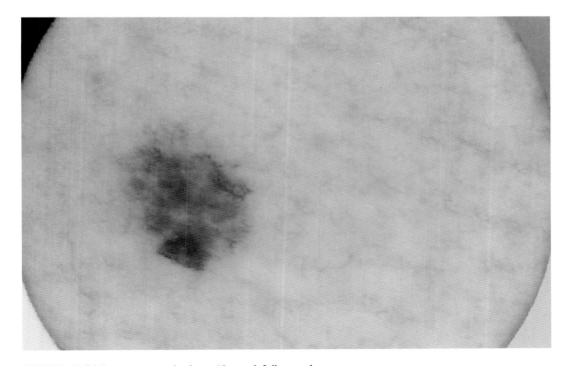

FIGURE 8.10 (b) Long-term monitoring—12 month follow-up image
Again ocal increase in pigmentation is more indicative that the lesion is melanoma. Diagnosis: 0.3 mm Breslow thick melanoma.

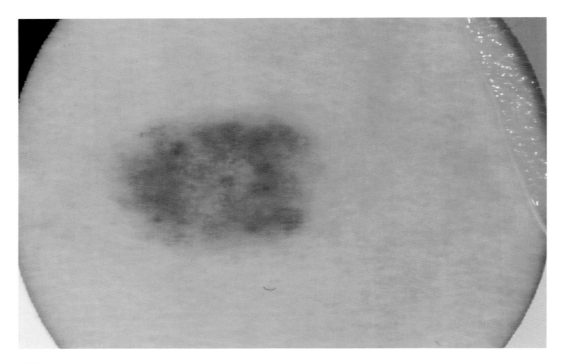

FIGURE 8.11 (a) Long-term monitoring—baseline image

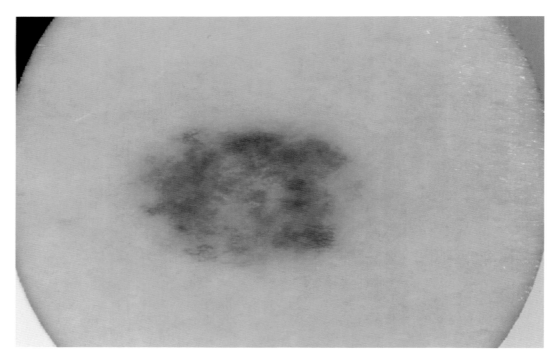

FIGURE 8.11 (b) Long-term monitoring—6 month follow-up image
Unlike 75% of melanomas, which when enlarge over long-term monitoring do so asymmetrically, this lesion has increased in size symmetrically. Note also the multiple internal architectural changes seen. Diagnosis: In situ melanoma.

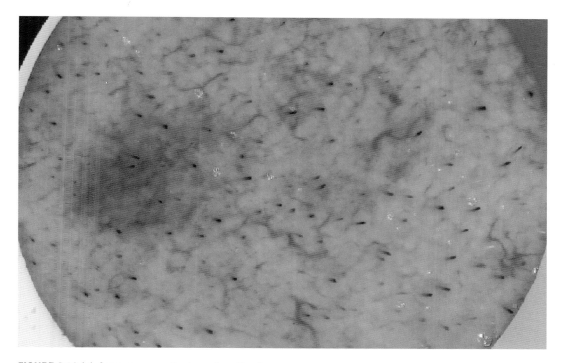

FIGURE 8.12 (a) Long-term monitoring—baseline image

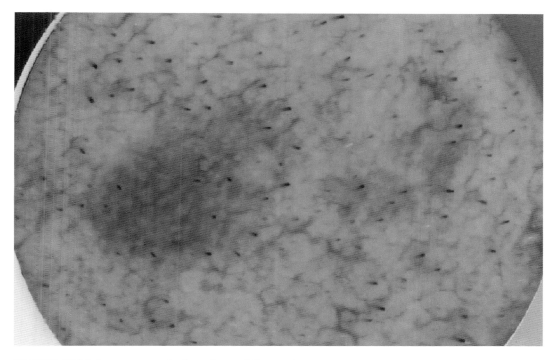

FIGURE 8.12 (b) Long-term monitoring—2 year follow-up image

This pigmented macule of the face underwent short-term (3 month) monitoring and was unchanged. However, long-term follow-up confirmed enlargement (albeit symmetrical). Only 75% of lentigo maligna will change over short-term (2.5–4.5 month) follow-up. When the diagnosis of lentigo maligna needs exclusion, it is recommended to repeat the monitoring between 6–12 months from the baseline image. Diagnosis: Lentigo maligna.

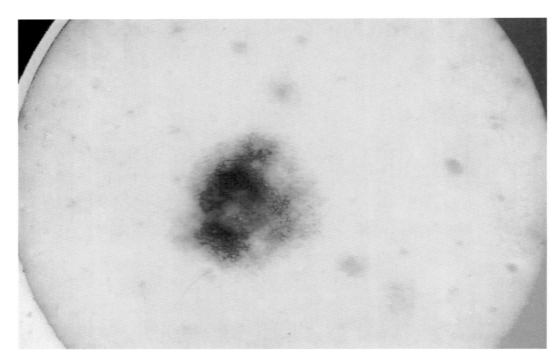

FIGURE 8.13 (a) Short-term monitoring—baseline image

In contrast to long-term monitoring, lesions that are suspicious but lack dermoscopy evidence of melanoma can be monitored over the relatively short time period of 3 months (range 2.5–4.5 months).

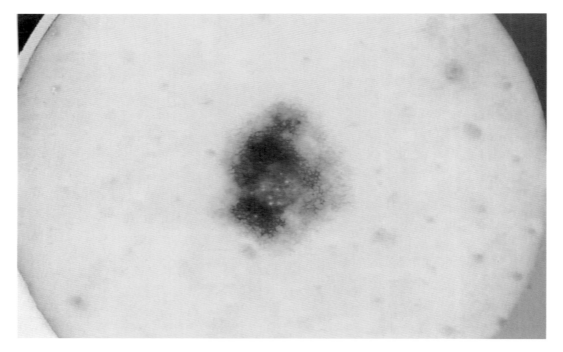

FIGURE 8.13 (b) Short-term monitoring—3 month follow-up image

In contrast to long-term monitoring any change over the short-term period (up to 4.5 months) is considered an indication to excise the lesion. The exceptions to this are an increase or decrease in milia-like cysts (as seen here), diffuse decrease or increase in pigmentation without architectural change (solar change), or an increase in size of nevi with multiple peripheral brown globules, or features indicating the lesion is a Spitz nevus.

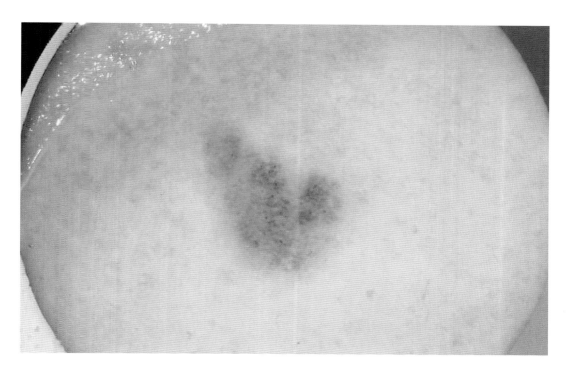

FIGURE 3.14 (a) Short-term monitoring—baseline image

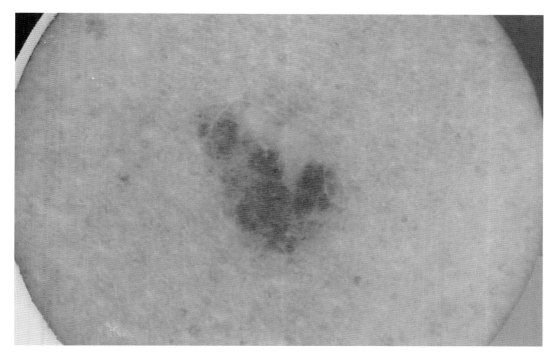

FIGURE 8.14 (b) Short-term monitoring—3 month follow-up image

In the case of the insignificant short-term change due to sun exposure (solar change), diffuse pigmentation change of the normal surrounding skin (tanning or lightening of the skin) usually parallels the changes seen within the lesion. However, the existing architecture remains the same (as seen here). It should also be noted that sun exposure can induce increased irregularity in nevi over the short-term monitoring period. To avoid incorrect interpretation of monitored changes, patients should avoid direct sun exposure of their monitored nevi.

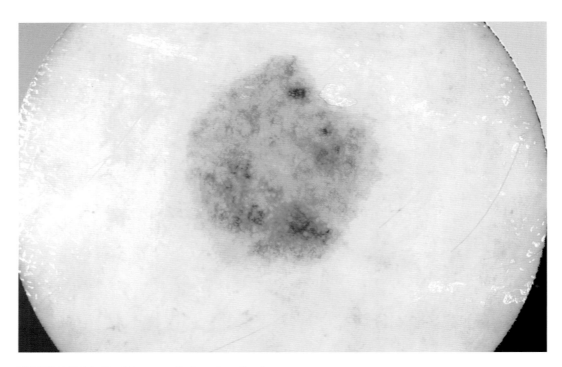

FIGURE 8.15 (a) Short-term monitoring—baseline image

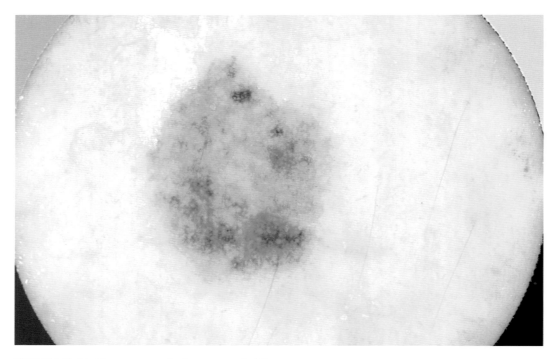

FIGURE 8.15 (b) Short-term monitoring—3 month follow-up image

Sometimes stretching of a lesion can induce a pseudo-change. However, this is usually easily seen as elongation along one axis with a corresponding decreased width of the perpendicular axis. Here no change is seen on follow-up. Of lesions unchanged at short-term follow-up, 99.2% are benign.

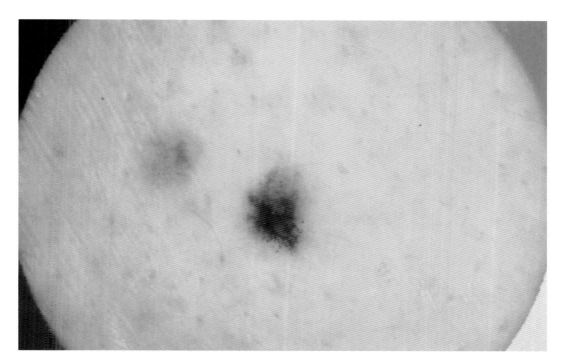

FIGURE 8.16 (a) Short-term monitoring—baseline image

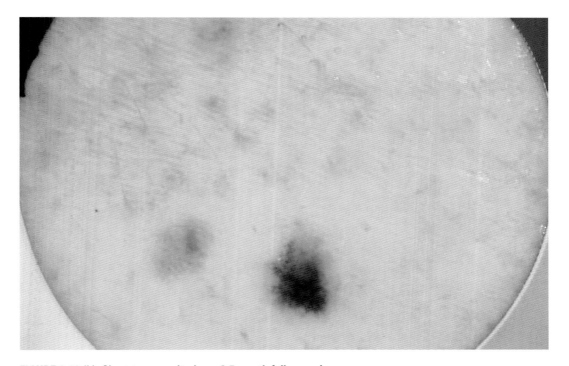

FIGURE 8.16 (b) Short-term monitoring—3.5 month follow-up image
Here the lesion has changed shape, distribution of brown globules at one pole and has some subtle color change centrally.
Diagnosis: Superficial spreading melanoma 0.25 mm Breslow depth.

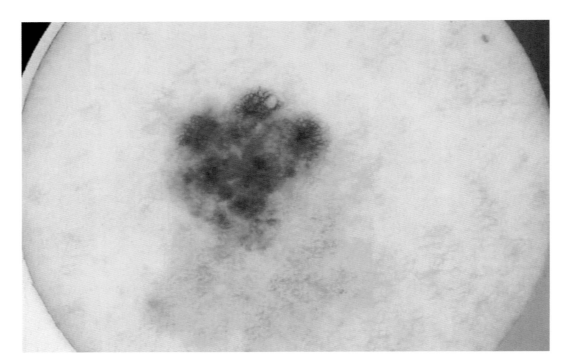

FIGURE 8.17 (a) Short-term monitoring—baseline image

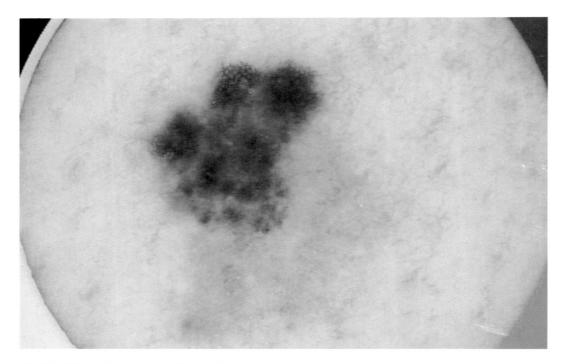

FIGURE 8.17 (b) Short-term monitoring—3 month follow-up image
Here there is a dramatic increase in size of the darker pigmented component of the lesion. Diagnosis: Superficial spreading melanoma 0.3 mm Breslow depth.

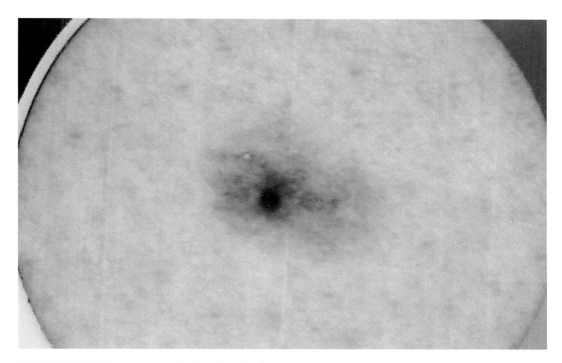

FIGURE 8.18 (a) Short-term monitoring—baseline image

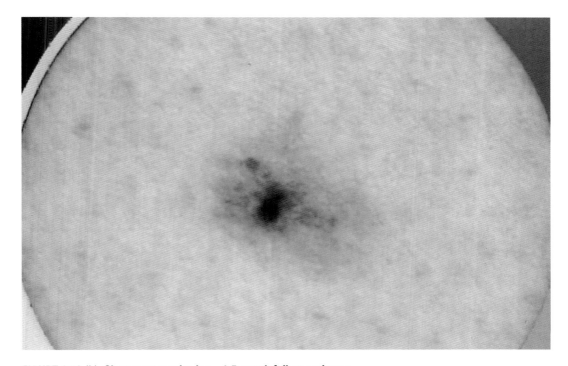

FIGURE 8.18 (b) Short-term monitoring—1.5 month follow-up image
Here the central dark focus has changed (increased width of projection). Note the short monitoring period in this case. While two-thirds of melanomas change at 6 weeks of monitoring, one-third require the full interval of 2.5–4.5 months before changes are seen. For this reason we advise 3 months (within 2.5–4.5 months) as the standard monitoring period for short-term surveillance of suspicious melanocytic lesions. Ninety four percent of melanoma (non-lentigo maligna type) will change at this time. Diagnosis: Focal invasive melanoma 0.28 mm Breslow depth arising in a compound dysplastic nevus.

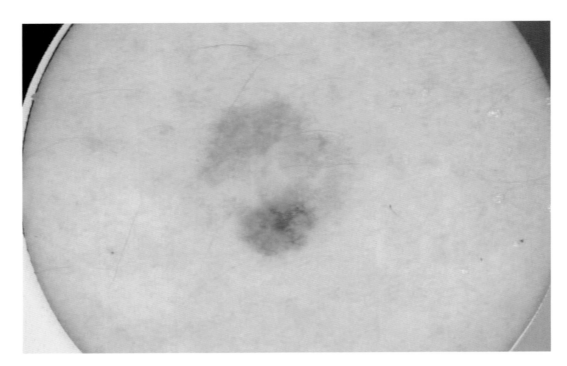

FIGURE 8.19 (a) Short-term monitoring—baseline image

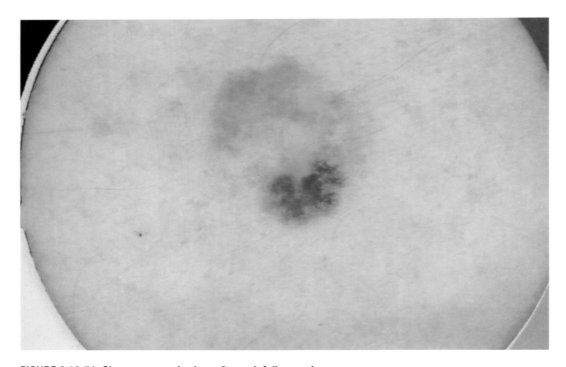

FIGURE 8.19 (b) Short-term monitoring—3 month follow-up image

Here the dark focus of the lesion has increased in size. Diagnosis: Focal in situ melanoma arising in a compound dysplastic nevus.

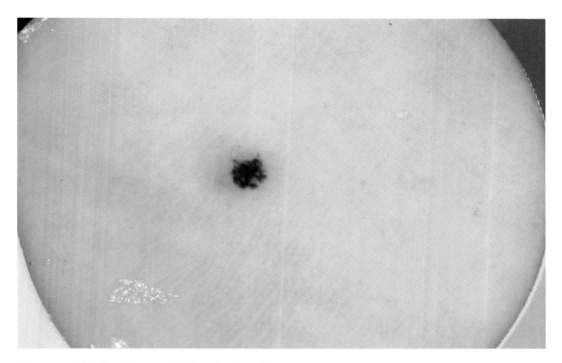

FIGURE 8.20 (a) Short-term monitoring—baseline image

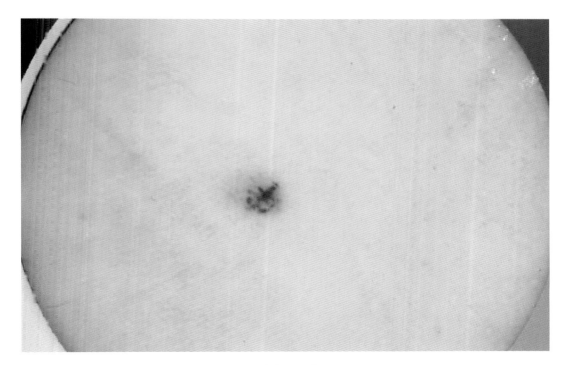

FIGURE 8.20 (b) Short-term monitoring—3 month follow-up image
This rapidly changing 2 mm diameter lesion shows significant depigmentation. It should be emphasized that some melanomas have a less atypical appearance following monitoring (see also Figure 8.16). Hence, with short-term monitoring, the finding of a more "benign" appearance still requires excision biopsy. Diagnosis: In situ melanoma.

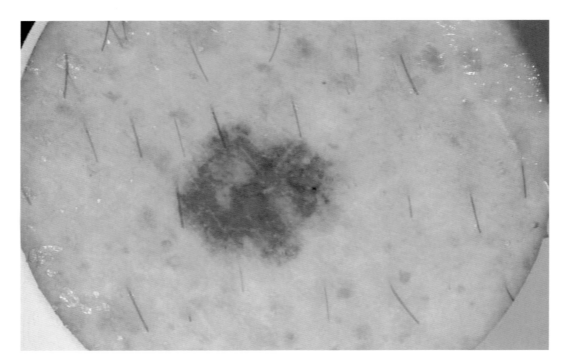

FIGURE 8.21 (a) Short-term monitoring—baseline image

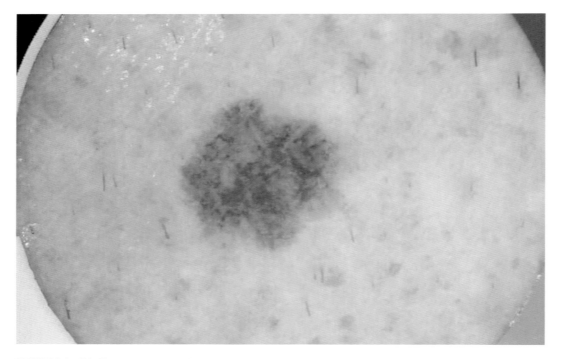

FIGURE 8.21 (b) Short-term monitoring—3 month follow-up image
Here subtle changes in architecture occur scattered throughout the lesion. While there is also solar change in this monitored lesion the changes in architecture require excision biopsy. Diagnosis: In situ melanoma.

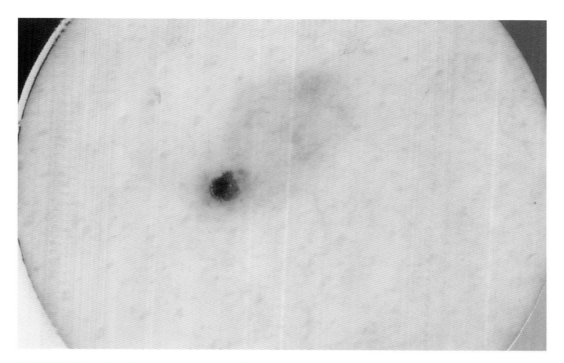

FIGURE 8.22 (a) Short-term monitoring—baseline image

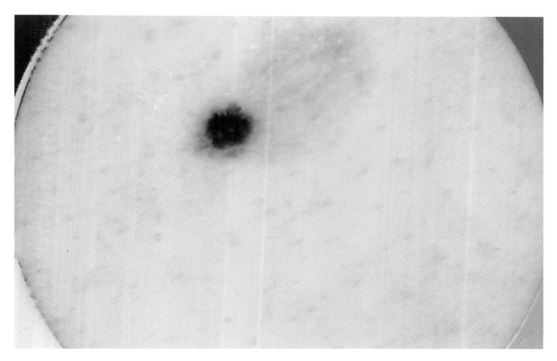

FIGURE 8.22 (b) Short-term monitoring—4 month follow-up image
Diagnosis: In situ melanoma.

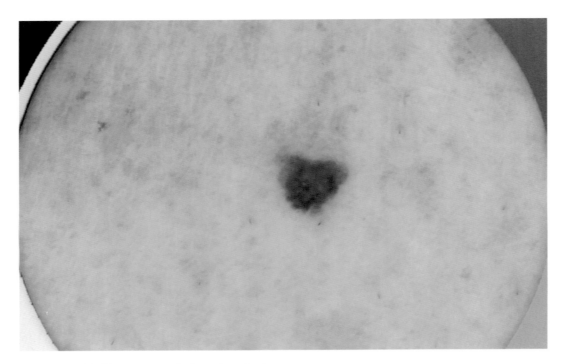

FIGURE 8.23 (a) Short-term monitoring—baseline image

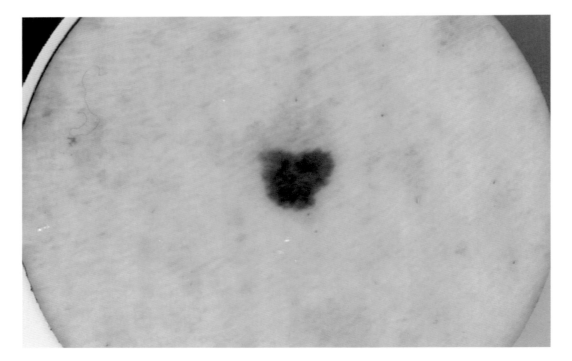

FIGURE 8.23 (b) Short-term monitoring—4 month follow-up image

Here the lesion has increased in size with architectural change within the lesion. Unlike long-term monitoring there is no particular type of change that predicts melanoma versus benign changes in short-term monitoring. For this reason all changing lesions must be excised. Diagnosis: In situ melanoma.

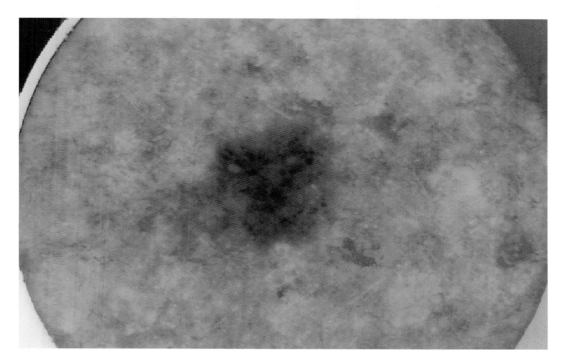

FIGURE 8.24 (a) Short-term monitoring—baseline image

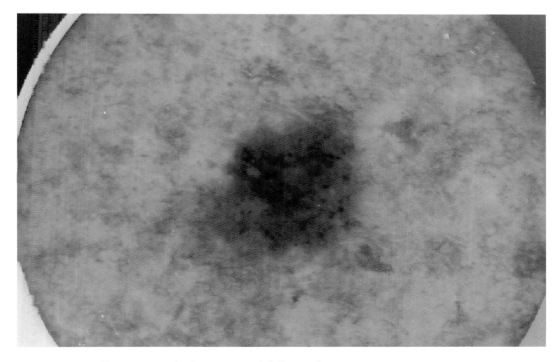

FIGURE 8.24 (b) Short-term monitoring—2.5 month follow-up image
Diagnosis: In situ melanoma.

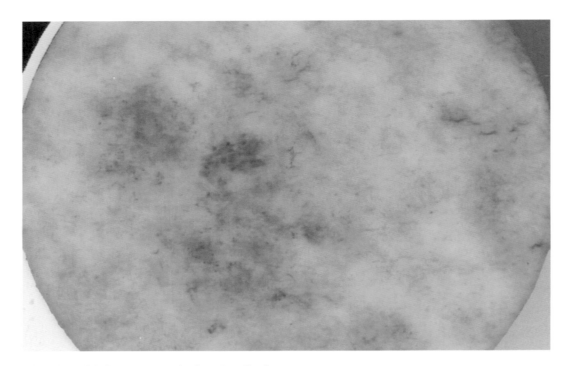

FIGURE 8.25 (a) Short-term monitoring—baseline image

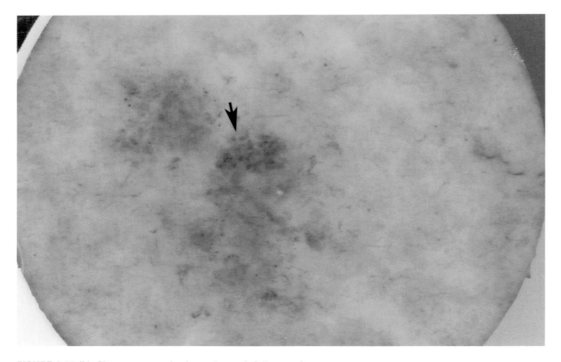

FIGURE 8.25 (b) Short-term monitoring—4 month follow-up image
Definite but subtle change occurred in this lesion (arrow). Diagnosis: 0.3 mm Breslow thick melanoma.

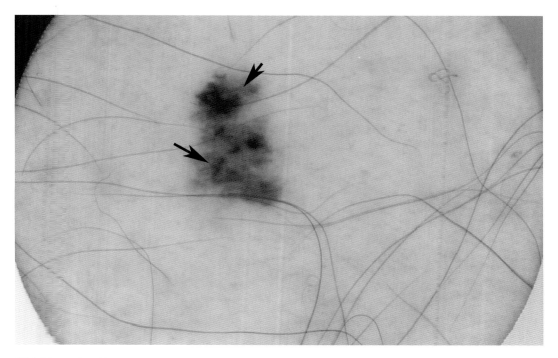

FIGURE 8.26 (a) Short-term monitoring—baseline image

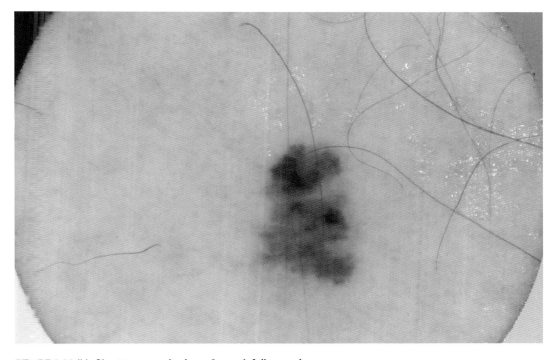

FIGURE 8.26 (b) Short-term monitoring—3 month follow-up image
The arrows in the baseline image indicates the internal architectural change (loss of pigmentation). Diagnosis: 0.35 mm Breslow thick superficial spreading melanoma.

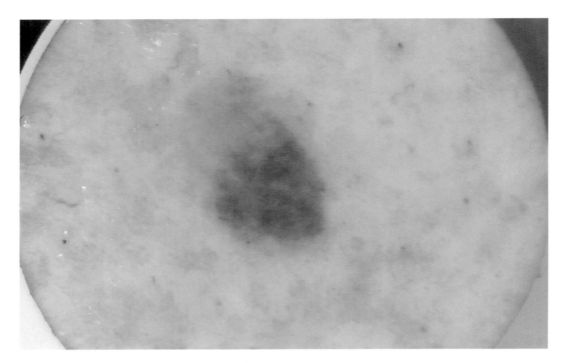

FIGURE 8.27 (a) Short-term monitoring—baseline image

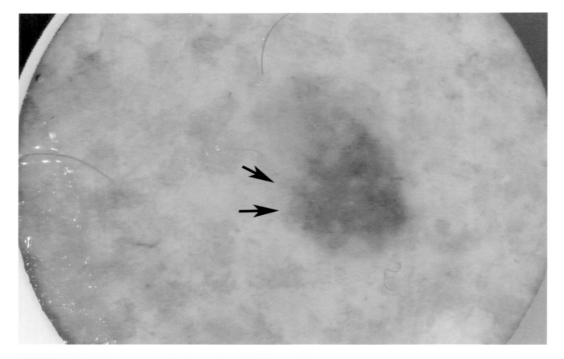

FIGURE 8.27 (b) Short-term monitoring—3 month follow-up image
The arrows indicate the focal increase in size and internal architectural change of the lesion. Diagnosis: In situ melanoma.

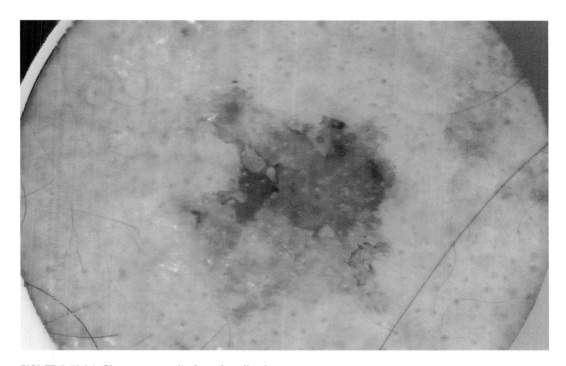

FIGURE 8.28 (a) Short-term monitoring—baseline image
This lesion on the scalp has the appearance of an ephelis with a moth-eaten edge and uniform pigment background.

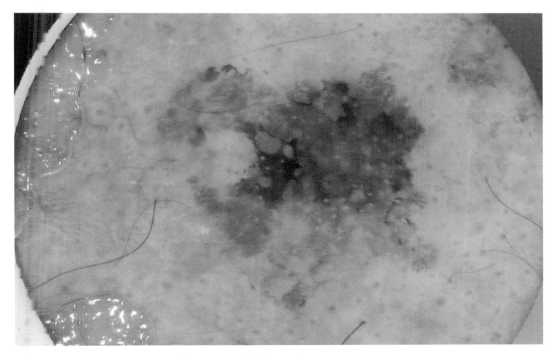

FIGURE 8.28 (b) Short-term monitoring—3 month follow-up image
The dramatic increase in size is noted. Diagnosis: Lentigo maligna.

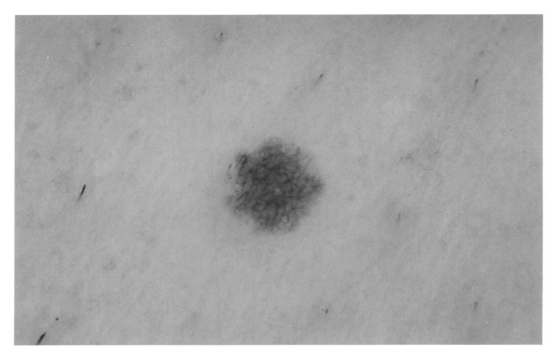

FIGURE 8.29 (a) New and changing lesion on the leg of a 38-year-old woman

The advantage of short-term monitoring is that lesions that would normally be observed, such as this dermoscopically banal lesion, can be monitored in an appropriate clinical setting. This 2.5 mm diameter lesion on the anterior tibia was noted to be new and changing by a 38-year-old woman. Under dermoscopic examination it is seen as a symmetrical lesion with graduated network at the periphery. However, because of the history of change the lesion was monitored.

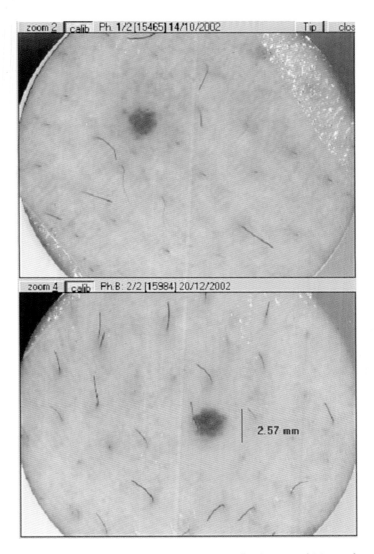

FIGURE 8.29 (b) Short-term monitoring—baseline image and 2.5 month follow-up image

Here the lesion has clearly enlarged over the short-term follow-up. Diagnosis: In situ melanoma. Nearly two-thirds of melanomas detected by short-term monitoring lack specific dermoscopic features of melanoma.

CHAPTER NINE

SUMMARY

Melanocytic lesion

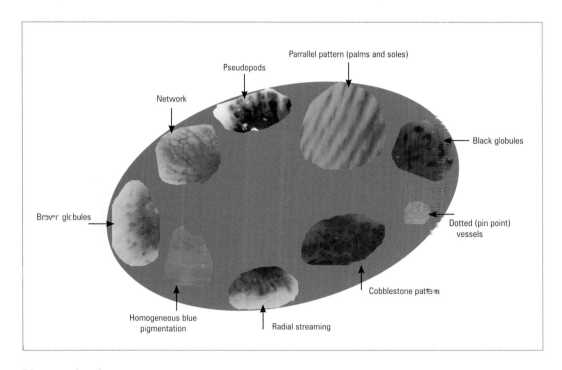

Pigmented melanoma

Asymmetric pattern and more than one colour

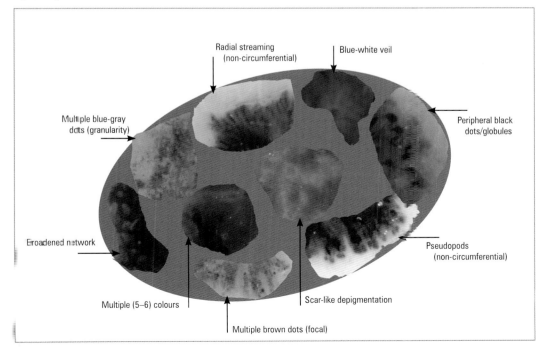

Amelanotic/hypomelanotic melanoma
Additional features to pigmented melanoma

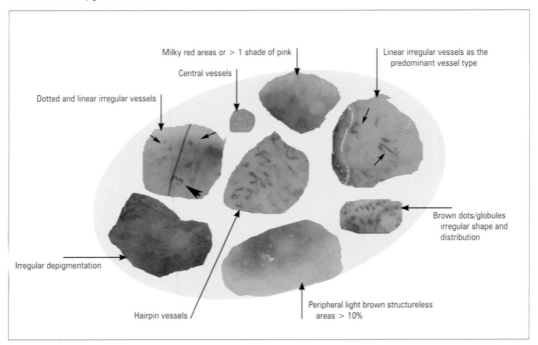

Milky red areas or > 1 shade of pink

Central vessels

Dotted and linear irregular vessels

Linear irregular vessels as the predominant vessel type

Brown dots/globules irregular shape and distribution

Irregular depigmentation

Hairpin vessels

Peripheral light brown structureless areas > 10%

Lentigo maligna
Additional features to other melanoma

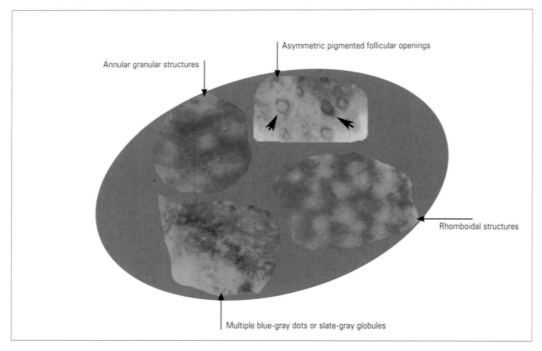

Asymmetric pigmented follicular openings

Annular granular structures

Rhomboidal structures

Multiple blue-gray dots or slate-gray globules

Acral melanoma

More than 7mm with lack of regular parallel furrow/lattice or fibrillar patterns. Additional features to other melanomas

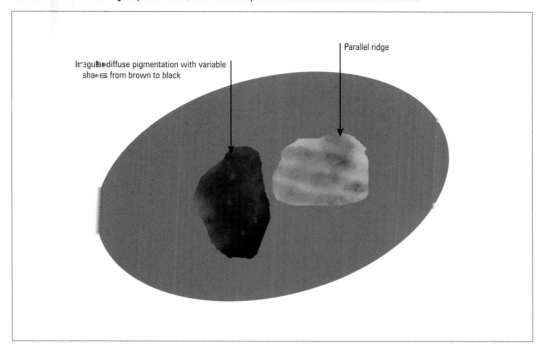

Irregular diffuse pigmentation with variable shades from brown to black

Parallel ridge

Epidermis/solar lentigo

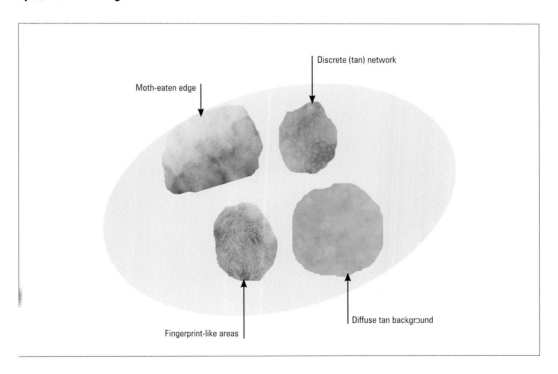

Moth-eaten edge

Discrete (tan) network

Fingerprint-like areas

Diffuse tan background

Banal acquired nevi
Usually symmetrical pattern

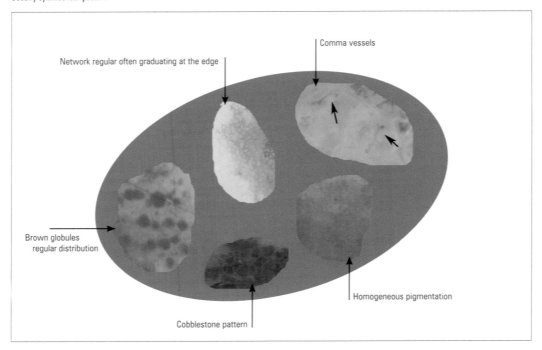

Network regular often graduating at the edge

Comma vessels

Brown globules regular distribution

Cobblestone pattern

Homogeneous pigmentation

Dysplastic nevi
Often asymmetric pattern

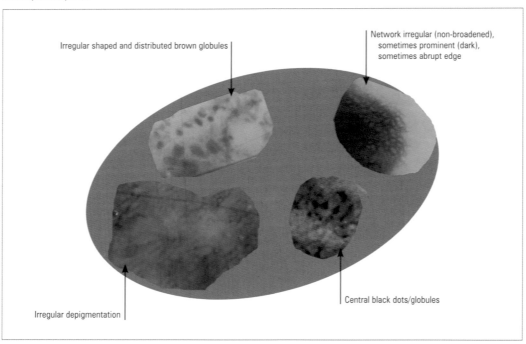

Irregular shaped and distributed brown globules

Network irregular (non-broadened), sometimes prominent (dark), sometimes abrupt edge

Irregular depigmentation

Central black dots/globules

Spitz nevi
Usually symmetrical pattern

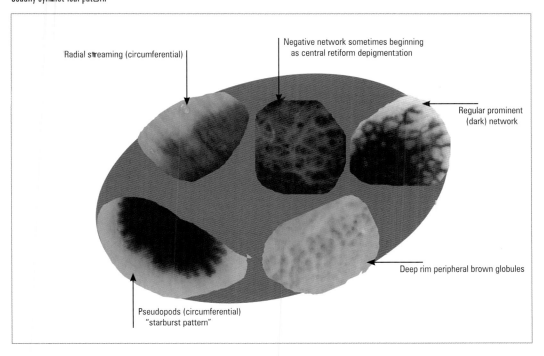

Radial streaming (circumferential)

Negative network sometimes beginning as central retiform depigmentation

Regular prominent (dark) network

Deep rim peripheral brown globules

Pseudopods (circumferential) "starburst pattern"

Pigmented BCC
No pigment network

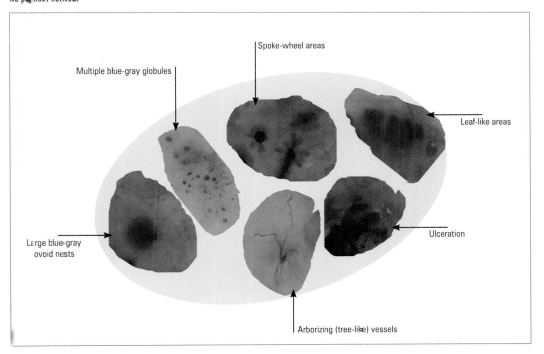

Multiple blue-gray globules

Spoke-wheel areas

Leaf-like areas

Large blue-gray ovoid nests

Ulceration

Arborizing (tree-like) vessels

Hemangioma

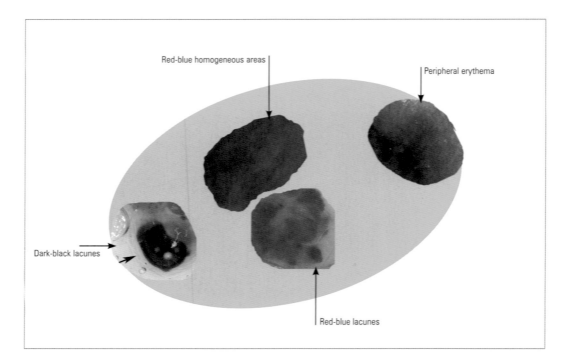

Red-blue homogeneous areas

Peripheral erythema

Dark-black lacunes

Red-blue lacunes

Seborrheic keratosis

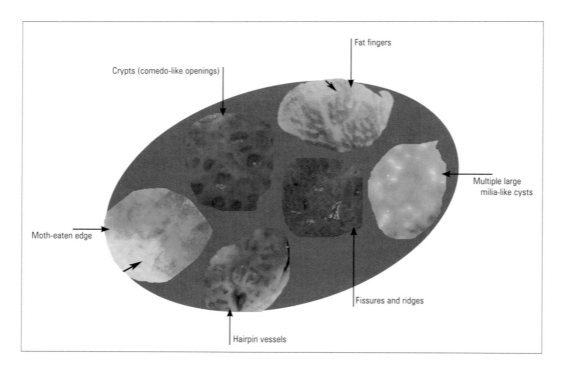

Fat fingers

Crypts (comedo-like openings)

Multiple large milia-like cysts

Moth-eaten edge

Fissures and ridges

Hairpin vessels

Dermatofibroma

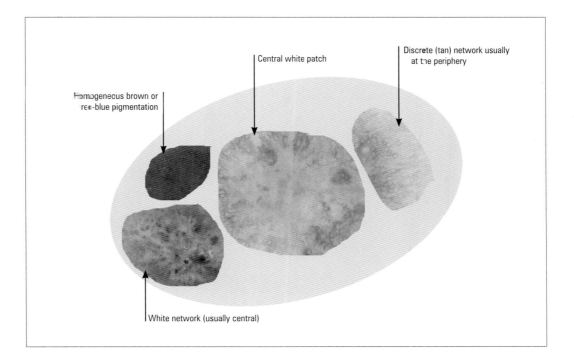

Central white patch

Discrete (tan) network usually at the periphery

Homogeneous brown or red-blue pigmentation

White network (usually central)